SO MUCH TO

Smile

ABOUT

SO MUCH TO

Smile

ABOUT

Transformational Dentistry
For a Younger, Healthier You

DRS. JULIE MARSHALL & DOUG BAXTER

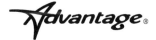

Published by Advantage, Charleston, South Carolina.
Member of Advantage Media Group.

ADVANTAGE is a registered trademark and the Advantage colophon is a trademark of Advantage Media Group, Inc.

Printed in the United States of America.

ISBN: 978-1-59932-489-0
LCCN: 2015950101

This publication is designed to provide accurate and authoritative information in regard to the subject matter covered. It is sold with the understanding that the publisher is not engaged in rendering legal, accounting, or other professional services. If legal advice or other expert assistance is required, the services of a competent professional person should be sought.

Advantage Media Group is proud to be a part of the Tree Neutral® program. Tree Neutral offsets the number of trees consumed in the production and printing of this book by taking proactive steps such as planting trees in direct proportion to the number of trees used to print books. To learn more about Tree Neutral, please visit www.treeneutral.com. To learn more about Advantage's commitment to being a responsible steward of the environment, please visit www.advantagefamily.com/green

Advantage Media Group is a publisher of business, self-improvement, and professional development books and online learning. We help entrepreneurs, business leaders, and professionals share their Stories, Passion, and Knowledge to help others Learn & Grow. Do you have a manuscript or book idea that you would like us to consider for publishing? Please visit advantagefamily.com or call 1.866.775.1696.

Dedicated to our family,
Duard and Dorothy Baxter and Dee Russell,
for their constant support and encouragement.
We love you.

CONTENTS

INTRODUCTION

As sibling owners of Total Transformation Dental and Spa, we—Julie and Doug—work together in the same building in which our father started a dentistry practice on Broad Street in Winder, Georgia.

It was "bread-and-butter" dentistry, with our father, Dr. D.O. Baxter, already in business for 30 years before we came onboard. Although people even then didn't really like coming to the dentist, they loved coming to visit our father in his practice. He was well known for being very gentle, and we saw patients constantly bringing him thoughtful gifts—cakes and other foodstuffs.

Our mom, Dorothy Baxter, was the hygienist in the practice, and our parents were very happy and well liked in the community. In fact, after seeing how happy our parents were, we wanted the same for ourselves.

So after dental school, we followed in our father's footsteps, starting practices in the same building where he practiced. Our sister, Dee Russell had already completed hygiene school and was practicing as a full time hygienist in our father's practice. Dr. Marshall joined the practice in 1988 and Dr. Baxter in 1992.

We never envisioned a dentistry practice like we have now. But dentistry has changed so much. We now see the benefits of the newest products and techniques and also an evolution in what patients want.

Surprisingly, our state-of-the-art practice has thrived in a very small town, a testament to the possibilities that exist in today's marketplace. We never envisioned having the range that the practice now offers. Some of the things we do now weren't done anywhere back when it was just our father in practice.

Advances offered at the practice today include Botox, which helps with pain management for patients who are chronic clenchers and grinders. The Botox relaxes the muscles involved in clenching, releasing the pressure that creates tension headaches and other associated issues such as wearing of the teeth and damage to the jaw joint. This is a prime example of the evolution of dentistry. Today it's about more than just teeth—it's also about the surrounding structures that allow people to smile, eat, and talk.

When our father was practicing, it was very common to take out teeth. In today's practice, with so many advances available, extractions are rare, and teeth are more commonly saved: there are better ways to combat decay, periodontal disease, and other problems through preventive measures that didn't exist generations ago.

Beyond dental school, we've both learned about preventive measures through continuing education—learning not just to treat diseases of the mouth but also to understand and deal with some of the underlying factors that can cause problems. These include the effects of medications on the mouth and risk factors such as diabetes and smoking.

The transformational model that our practice now offers began when, over time, we decided we wanted to add services to what we were already offering.

It all started with Julie attending a course offered by the American Academy of Facial Esthetics, a fairly intense training series ending in a certification for Botox and dermal filler. Julie had seen an advertisement for the course in a dental journal when the process was still unapproved in Georgia.

As part of the course, attendees performed the techniques on each other, and Julie was amazed at the results and excited at what esthetics could do for dentistry.

Patients were already coming to the practice because they trusted us with their dental needs, so the transformation of the practice to include other services that enhance facial features was just a natural progression. The process was approved in Georgia in December 2013, and because Julie had already been spreading the word with longtime patients, we already had a patient waiting for treatment as soon as she was certified.

That first patient trusted us implicitly, as have others who have since taken advantage of the services. Since then, our practice has added facials, peels, and waxing to its offerings and is the only practice in the area with these services.

The evolution of the practice mirrors the change in attitudes toward appearances over time. When our father was in dental school, fillings were composed of the silver-colored amalgam filling, gold, or—near the end of his time in practice—early versions of composite and porcelain. He basically had very limited materials to use, and we can remember what an exciting time it was when we were first able to use a natural tooth-colored filling; it was a huge breakthrough.

Today, there are a dozen different types of composite materials and different types of porcelain that we can use on certain restorations.

There have been other breakthroughs over the years. Take whitening, for example. Twenty years ago, teeth whitening was performed rarely and then only by a qualified dentist in an office. Today, toothpastes and rinses are regularly advertised in all forms of media. This demonstrates how people want their teeth to not only function properly but to look nice as well.

In fact, a number of new faces have become patients in our practice just for the cosmetic procedures. And patients who have put off recommended dental procedures for years are now having those done following a good experience on the esthetic side of the practice. Those facial esthetics, we've found, give a bit of self-confidence—a boost toward patients taking better care of themselves overall.

In essence, giving patients what they want has encouraged them to listen to us and trust us to help them with what they need. And the total transformation of the practice means that patients can have everything for the face done in one place by someone they trust.

Today, patients can transform their dental health while enhancing their physical appearance. We, meanwhile, are receiving instant gratification for our training and dedication. It's an exciting time at Total Transformation Dental and Spa.

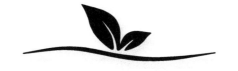

Chapter One

HOW WE BECAME A TOTAL TRANSFORMATION PRACTICE

People are surprised to learn about our practice, since it combines dentistry with facial rejuvenation techniques.

Often, their first reaction is, "Have you ever done this before?" Their belief is that Botox is a procedure performed by dermatologists; they don't see it as a dental procedure. And that surprises us; we think it should be in our ballpark, since we deal with the face all day anyway. We just feel like it's a natural transition for us to be injecting outside of the mouth, since we also do injections inside the mouth.

In fact, during training it became apparent to us that we had a leg up on the idea of combining both dental and esthetics, as we were called upon to do the inside-the-mouth shots for physicians and other medical professionals who were having trouble with the procedure. We didn't have to relearn all the facial muscles, because we do this sort of injecting every day.

In truth, we face a more challenging biological landscape; we have to do a lot of blind injections because veins in the mouth and arteries are invisible to the naked eye. We have to rely on landmarks in a patient's mouth and on the face; we have to know where those muscles are, their function, and how they contract, so that we can know what to expect when we inject the anesthetic or Botox. When you're getting a shot in the arm, that's a large muscle—it's hard to miss that muscle. But on the face there are muscles that overlap other muscles. We have to make sure we're stopping that needle in the more superficial muscle, if that's where we need it, versus penetrating it and going into the one underneath it.

For instance, when you're doing a gummy smile treatment—for patients who show too much gum tissue when they smile—you have to hit a certain muscle to keep the lip from coming up. If you go too deep, you're going to hit the muscle that's going to give an undesired result and could even cause the lip to droop, which would be the total opposite of what you're trying to accomplish. That's a blind injection with Botox.

Our training with anesthesia trained us for this. For instance, to work on the mandible—the lower teeth—you have to give a nerve block that blocks the whole side. We have to go all the way back behind the teeth, up the ramus bone, and we have to determine where the nerve is. So we have to know bony and soft-tissue landmarks, and we have to be able to palpate certain areas, locating the nerve by touch—there's not a red pencil in there showing us where the nerve is. And we've been giving these shots for decades.

MASTERS OF PAIN MANAGEMENT

Pain-free dentistry has become a primary focus in dentistry.

Keeping the patient comfortable during dental procedures is paramount, and ensuring that they are appropriately numb before beginning is of the utmost importance in that equation.

Time was, the dentist started with a bit of topical anesthetic to numb the gum followed by a shot of Novocain. Today, there are topical anesthetics available that are different than anything in the past. It used to be that the dentist would place the topical in the mouth at the site of the injection and leave it in a few minutes to promote numbness. But topical anesthetics these days are much stronger, and they feel dry. The dentist places the topical in the mouth, and it stays a lot longer.

Handpieces—or the delivery systems—are also different today. They're measured and faster so that it doesn't take as long to do the procedure. Needles are different sizes; they're finer and available in different lengths and diameters.

These advances—along with the skilled, steady hands of trained and experienced doctors of dentistry—make the anesthesia process virtually pain-free for the patient. The result is a more sophisticated numbing process that doesn't leave patients feeling like there's a giant numb balloon on the side of their face.

Our skill as dentists translates into more than comfort during dental procedures; it also produces safe and superior results when it comes to injectable facial rejuvenation techniques such as Botox and fillers. Conversely, physicians—medical doctors—who aren't skilled in these procedures can't keep up with patients' demands these days.

We really see it going back to the issue of trust. Today, when the dentist says, "This won't hurt a bit," it's essentially true. We admit that we're reluctant when it comes to injections, so for us it's a matter of "doing unto others." We know that the dental office chair, "The Big Chair," as it's known, is the most intimidating seat in the house.

So our goal is to eliminate that fearful feeling, starting with the first visit. It's a learned trust that is built by getting to know the patient. Our team really wants to learn what we can about the patient as a person—it's more than just the patient's mouth, medical history, and current problems. It's a lesson we learned from our father: there's a person attached to that mouth, and that's who's being treated—not just teeth, not just a mouth.

Our practice also promotes a sense of ease, with soft music and essential oil diffusers in every room. It's a welcoming, comforting environment, whether a patient is coming in for a dental or esthetic procedure. We also find it to be a relaxing environment to work in.

ARCHITECTS OF
THE FACE

In addition to being artists at injections, we are architects of the entire face.

The teeth, jaws, and associated tissues—gums, muscles, and ligaments—provide the underlying support structure of the face. Tooth problems and bone loss play into an aged appearance that is literally more than skin deep.

Our superior knowledge of the facial structures provides superior results for patients when it comes to personal appearance. A person can go to a dermatologist or esthetic surgeon to get a facelift, but we know that real beauty is more than skin deep—it starts with a healthy underlying structure.

Everything is connected—the teeth, the jaw, the face—everything. An unhealthy structure makes all the difference. For example, people who are missing teeth and don't replace them may experience a shrunken facial structure and drooping features. Missing teeth in the back of the mouth can tremendously age a person; who hasn't seen someone age by years once they removed their dentures? Or consider how significant jaw problems can lead to grinding the teeth down. Problems with the jaw can also lead to a swollen, enlarged masseter muscle on the side of the face.

The appearance of the gums is another piece of the esthetics puzzle. Gums that are red, puffy, swollen, or off-color are unattractive and can throw off the entire face. But we can look at the appearance of the gums and their relationship to the lips and tell immediately what needs to be done.

Expertise in these areas has allowed us to develop a practice model that we call the "total transformation," because it pairs state-of-the art dental and facial rejuvenation techniques to transform not only our patients' smiles but their total look.

PROVEN RESULTS

It's a practice model with proven results, and we have the testimonials to prove that.

"I have to voice that I was so afraid of going to the dentist. I had let it go too long. Then due to extreme pain I broke down and had to go. I met Melissa (I call her my angel), she even cried with me and let me know that I can get my dental health back. And even be able to smile! I was given a plan by Dr. Baxter. He worked with me! I owe them so much. If you are looking for a family dentist, I suggest you try them. They are here for you 24 hours a day. Who else can say that?"
—Sandy P.

"I really am glad to not have the fear like I had to start out with. I want the dentist to be just another place I feel comfortable going to."
—Barbara H.

"Everyone was absolutely amazing. I would definitely refer everyone I know to your office. Best experience at a dentist ever. I received bad news about my dental health that upset me immensely, but your staff was very comforting. I thank you so much for your willingness to work with me about the finances on my next visit. Without help with a payment plan I would not have any options except to keep suffering with the pain. Thanks again for everything!"
—Donna E.

"You guys are great! In all the years I've been coming to you, you have been pleasant, polite, professional, and, dare I say, even enjoyable, which is a bit funny when talking about a visit to the dentist office. There is not one thing about your practice that I would change."
—Hugh C.

Often, people who come in for their first dental appointment say they're just price shopping for other services, but usually that's not the case. They're checking out the practice—checking out the dentist or the office space. They're usually somewhat meek and mild, not even looking us in the face or eyes.

But once they've had their first treatment—especially some of the transformation treatments—they are totally different.

For example, a patient may come in for a cleaning, and at that time, we'll talk to them about what a good candidate they'd be for a whitening. We may do a chair-side introduction to introduce them to the idea of other esthetic procedures, such as Juvéderm if they have issues on the outside of their mouth—for example, if the corners of their mouth are drooping.

After one or two procedures, they're transformed into smiling, self-confident individuals with a newfound enjoyment of life. For instance, no one misses the two-week follow-up to check results following a Botox treatment, because they're so excited, and they want to have their picture taken. And the recall appointments are never missed either; everyone comes in right as scheduled for their three-month follow-up Botox.

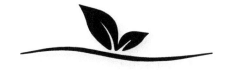

Chapter Two

GOOD ORAL HEALTH: THE FOUNDATION OF YOUTH

B y definition, just what is dentistry?

It's all about health. The gum tissue has to be healthy. The mouth needs to be decay free. The teeth need to function correctly, which means they need to be in the right position.

As the teeth come together, the ultimate goal is for everything around the arch, from the back to the front, to function normally when the patient bites down. One tooth should not take more of the brunt or more pressure than any others, because that will create problems. The overall health is the goal right from the start.

Oral health is crucial because if your mouth isn't healthy, you're not healthy. For instance, the same bugs and bacteria that we deal with when it comes to periodontal disease have a direct link to heart disease. Just like the plaque that builds up in the arteries, plaque also builds up on the teeth; it's not the same plaque, but there is a direct link.

If plaque stays in the mouth too long, gum tissue gets inflamed. And if there is inflammation anywhere in the body and it stays too long, you have to worry about infection. Take, for example, a wound outside the mouth, let's say, a child's scraped knee that has scabbed over, but then the child keeps scratching at the scab, which keeps it irritated and inflamed. If it stays irritated long enough, it provides an entryway for infection.

Now, the body tries hard to heal itself. When we take a tooth out, we'll tell the patient that one of the things to expect is a little bit of inflammation. That's normal. That's the body healing itself. An extraction is traumatic; it's a small trauma site. So anytime there is trauma, there's inflammation. The body sends inflammatory cells to a wounded or traumatized area, and that's where we get some of the healing.

However, infection slows down healing. For example, if someone comes into our office and has an abscessed tooth, we often have to deal with the infection first before we can do treatment. It depends on the amount of infection there is because infection also will not allow local anesthetic to work at 100 percent. If a patient has an abscessed tooth with a lot of swelling and the tooth has to come out, then we can't get the patient numb, and we don't want to try to get the tooth out.

We don't want the patient going through the experience of being uncomfortable. So there are other avenues we can use. We will put them on antibiotics sometimes to get rid of the infection, or sometimes we get the patient straight to the oral surgeon. There, the patient can be sedated first, and then the oral surgeon can get the tooth out even if it has considerable inflammation. Often, the oral surgeon has to drain the inflammation or the infection out before he can start, but he still has greater success where there's substantial inflammation.

Keeping the mouth clean and healthy keeps inflammation down and infection away.

MODERN DENTISTRY

Modern dentistry is devoted to saving natural teeth if at all possible. What God gave us is much better than anything man-made we can put in the mouth. Think about it: you see people out in public with crooked teeth—those teeth are angled and don't line up.

Even if there's no tooth decay, or if the teeth aren't in the right position, a person can deal with gum issues or periodontal disease. And over time, they can have a lot of uneven wear that creates problems for them down the road. Still, those teeth are much stronger than anything we can put in.

For example, angled teeth cause uneven wear and create problems in the jaw joint. Once a person starts chewing through the enamel in certain areas of the mouth, the teeth can become sensitive, or they can fracture or split, which of course creates discomfort.

If your teeth make it difficult to eat, you may not consume the correct foods; without the correct fuel, you're not helping your body overall. What we eat greatly affects how we feel and also our energy level. Anything we put in our mouths lowers the pH of our saliva, which creates an acidic environment. In this atmosphere, plaque turns into acid and damages the teeth.

So we need to eat healthy foods that keep our immune system strong but that also help us continue to grow properly and to maintain overall health throughout our lifetimes. All the healthy foods we're supposed to eat, such as fruits and vegetables, must be broken down small enough when you chew so that the rest of your system can digest them easily.

BUILDING A STRONG FOUNDATION

When we start a new patient relationship, we, of course, start with introductions. Then we look at the patient's medical history, including any issues of concern.

We use the terms "health" and "foundation" as part of the initial exam. Our ultimate goal is to have a very broad foundation—the teeth, the gums, and the bone—and to keep those healthy. Then everything builds on top of that.

Certainly, we're concerned if there's decay around the mouth, but we're more concerned if there's periodontal pocketing with the patient's gum tissue. But if the foundation is not healthy, the best restoration on a tooth won't do any good, because it just won't hold. It would be like putting very expensive shingles or a roof on a house that has a sagging foundation. If the foundation is not there, anything on top of it is going to be weak.

Where once cavities were the primary worry when it came to prevention, today we're seeing more links to periodontal disease because of what patients are putting in their bodies and some of the medicines that they take. Anything a person ingests can affect their overall health.

For example, if a patient is taking a long list of medications for everything from high blood pressure to cholesterol, it can greatly change their overall health, including the health of their mouth. Their health may not necessarily be going downhill, and they may have a very clean mouth, but they may not produce as much saliva as they used to. Without proper production of saliva, the mouth becomes more prone to decay because saliva is the lubricant that keeps plaque from sticking as much. Another example is diabetes. Diabetes is, of course, a chronic disease that has to be managed. Not only does it greatly affect the large organs of the body that all diabetics have to worry about, but it also causes gum issues and circulation issues, which are some of the other factors that we deal with.

The medical history that we take when we begin a relationship with a new patient addresses these chronic health concerns and associated medications. We want to review what they're taking and what conditions they have as they relate to the treatment they will receive from us. But what we've also discovered during this evaluation is that sometimes a patient has been taking so many medications for so long from different doctors that they don't even know why they're taking some of them. Sometimes, the medication was for an issue that has since been corrected, and on occasion, we find duplications from different prescribing doctors who are not in communication with each other.

For example, sometimes a person will be put on blood pressure medicine to correct a high blood pressure reading, but they've since improved their diet and begun a regular exercise program, which makes us question the need for the continuation of that medication.

Other times, a patient may come in with extremely elevated blood pressure, and we can't perform any services on them that day because of it; we don't want to mix anesthetic in with epinephrine if they're already on the top end of high blood pressure.

In short, sometimes a new patient's medical history involves a consultation with the patient's physician and other specialists.

It's interesting to watch patients gain a greater understanding of our true qualifications. They may think they've come in just to have a tooth looked at: "Doctor, it's just a tooth," they'll say. But with our medical expertise, we start by identifying other areas of concern.

So we tell patients: "It's just a tooth, but that tooth is connected to you. We've got to make sure you walk out of this building and you feel fine. We don't want to just work on a tooth, we want you coming back." We need to make sure anything we do is going to heal correctly. We have to manage not only the site that we're working in but also the patients themselves.

But sometimes they have had a laissez-faire attitude on certain teeth. "Just get it out, and all my problems will be gone," they think. Well, no. Sometimes taking teeth out creates other problems. It's a domino effect. Once we take out a tooth, we can't just leave a gaping hole there without repercussions.

For starters, the teeth will shift; if there's a tooth behind the one that's been pulled, it's going to drift forward. Teeth normally drift forward in the mouth anyway with age. The tooth above the missing space also looks for a match; it's looking for a mate to chew with, and it will continue to do so. It will slowly drop down and create a peri-odontal issue because it's changing the bones around the teeth, and it's changing the gum tissue. Eventually, it will make the space harder to clean as teeth line up into the contact area that is in between teeth that are being flossed. It sometimes creates a food catch, and it creates different wear patterns on other teeth.

So again, there are significant repercussions if you just take a tooth out and do nothing.

Make no mistake: we give patients options, one of which is to do nothing at all. But we explain that doing nothing is not a good option, because they obviously came to see us for a reason. They came to us for our opinion, so we give that to them. We will give them what we think are all their options, and then we try to help them decide what's best.

With the first appointment, and with all subsequent appointments, we do a blood pressure check on every patient. The first visit to the practice also includes an examination using advanced, patient-friendly technology such as, with permission, a digital X-ray that employs 98 percent less radiation. Other technologies include perio charting, which is a check of six sites on every tooth to examine the health of the gum tissue. We use an instrument called DIAGNO-dent, which is used on the tooth after the plaque is removed. The instrument is put on areas of a dry tooth—on the bite surface where there are pits and grooves. It uses light to determine tooth density and identify areas of decay.

New patients that visit our practice that aren't having problems also receive the same evaluation. For example, if a patient just moved to the area and they need a new dentist, we start with the same information to formulate a good starting point. We gather our own baseline information even if we have records that were sent from another dentist.

TREATMENT OF CAVITIES
AND DECAY

Everybody cringes when they hear the term "root canal."

That's why treatment of cavities and decay is so important, because these can progress to abscesses that cause infections requiring root canals.

Root canals have changed a lot over the years, but if you're dealing with infection, that is the cause of your pain. Removal of the nerve from the tooth under an anesthetic is literally a pain-free process. But if there's infection present and a lot of inflammation, that's where the trouble comes from.

For instance, a patient can have a root canal and even have it restored with a crown, but decay can still get below that crown—without cleaning, decay can get in. The tooth won't be sensitive because the root canal—removal of the nerve—took away the pain signal. There won't be any of the symptoms that would be present if the nerve was in the tooth. So a lot of times what we find is that the root canal masks a lot of issues.

That's why the X-rays are so important, so that we can see problems like that. When we tell a patient that he has a cavity in a root canal, inevitably he'll tell us he doesn't have any pain. And we always tell him how glad we are about that. "We're not looking for you to be in pain," we say, "but you've already invested money, time, and effort into restoring this tooth by having the root canal and the crown on it. Let's protect your investment and get the decay taken care of so that this tooth stays in your mouth and you can continue to use it."

Certainly, left unchecked, decay can lead to tooth loss, which can cause a domino effect like we mentioned earlier: teeth shifting, uneven wear, periodontal disease, and a food catch.

Recent studies have also shown a connection between the number of teeth a person loses and life longevity due to factors like nutrition and immunity. You're much healthier with a full complement of teeth.

Reiterating an earlier point: tooth loss also causes a more aged appearance.

Anytime a tooth comes out there's going to be some recession of bone. That starts immediately, because when the tooth comes out, it's a three-dimensional hole. It's not like a fracture in an arm; put a cast on that and it heals in six weeks. When a tooth is removed, that three-dimensional hole takes longer than six weeks to fill in. It does fill in over a period of months, but it will never have the same height and the same amount of bone that was there when the tooth was in. So the recession of the bone starts right when the extraction is done.

When a person loses a tooth, without the structure of that tooth in place, you also start seeing the collapse of facial structures. Some of the facial features in the cheeks or the lips literally fold into these areas. We see this all the time in patients with dentures. They have them in for a certain amount of time, and then they come in and tell us that their dentures don't fit like they used to. Well, the denture didn't change because acrylic doesn't change; instead, the structures underneath changed.

That bone continues to resorb unless it has something in the space, which is why an implant placed in the hole helps maintain bone. The implant is something for the bone to grow around, and it also more closely approximates the pressure of the natural tooth.

You've probably seen a picture of an elderly man who doesn't have any teeth, and when he doesn't have the dentures in, his nose almost touches his chin. He rolls his lips in, and he just completely collapses. That's a prime example of how the facial structures collapse. If he's collapsed down that far, think of the stress it's putting on his jaw joint. If you put that type of stress on your knees or on your elbows, you're dealing with discomfort.

The DIAGNOdent mentioned earlier helps identify tooth decay. It shoots a beam of light down onto the tooth and then reads the feedback as it reflects off the density of the tooth structure. The bounce-back of the light gives us the reading; a tooth with no decay will get a very low reading. The tool also has an audible sound to it, so as the numbers get higher, it makes a different noise, too.

The DIAGNOdent is only used to diagnose virgin teeth, which are teeth with no restorations; we use it to measure the density of a tooth with no fillings. We put it on the pits and grooves of the biting surface. That's the thinnest part of enamel even on a healthy tooth; it's a lot thinner than the thick and prominent cusp tip and a lot thinner than the side of the tooth.

It's an invaluable tool; we really couldn't practice without it. It allows us to diagnose decay at a very early stage.

When we do fillings that are caught at a very early stage, the patient doesn't even have to be numbed, because the damage is so small.

The treatment at that point is at the very surface of the tooth, allowing us to use a specific cone-shaped burr to remove the decay. We don't have to remove near as much tooth structure because the decay has just broken through the enamel. That's what constitutes a cavity—the plaque eats through the enamel and goes through that next layer of dentin. But if the decay is just at the surface, we can remove it with very minimal prepping—a lot of times we can do it without anesthetic.

By catching the damage early, there is much more tooth structure to support the filling. Again, having a lot of tooth structure is important—that's the only way to keep it in the filling range.

When the restoration goes from a filling to more of an onlay or a crown, there isn't enough tooth structure to support it. Once the fillings start getting larger and there isn't much tooth structure left, that's usually when the restoration of choice has to go from a filling to a crown.

Sometimes a patient comes in and we see a lot of stain on the tooth, but we won't get a high reading on the DIAGNOdent. But we know that if stain stays there long enough, it's just a matter of time before it's going to break through the dentin. So we'll open those grooves up a little bit to get the stain out so we can put a sealant on the tooth. That's not a filling but rather a sealant.

To reiterate, when the decay is minor enough, we don't have to anesthetize it as long as there is no discomfort for the patient. If we think that the area is minor, we'll tell the patient we don't believe there's a need to get them numb. We offer them the option to be numbed, but most of them decline. We tell them, "We'll get started. There's going to be water squirting on there, and if the water feels cold, if it makes the area too sensitive, or if anything that we're doing bothers you, motion with your hand and we'll stop. If we need to get you numb, we'll get you numb."

If the damage goes deeper—down into the dentin where it becomes a cavity—then we have to remove more of the tooth structure. In that case, we'll use a burr that has large grooves in it with a few cutting surfaces. The difference between the cone-shaped burr and the burr with large grooves is almost like the difference in teeth on different saw blades. A rough-cut saw has far fewer teeth, while a fine-cutting one has a lot of different, smaller teeth. The fine-cut type of burr is what we use on surface decay.

But if a filling is warranted, the process is much more comfortable today for the patient. The anesthetic part of filling a cavity is largely the same as it was decades ago, although the topical anesthetics are much more effective, and the injection techniques are more precise. Plus, the needles are better quality—they have a better beveled end, which gives a sharper point.

The silver amalgam, or metal, fillings are still relatively the same. The prep still has to undercut a lot of the tooth just to hold that filling in because it has to be held in with mechanical retention. But now we have bonded fillings, which are tooth colored. These are literally adhered to the tooth structure, and we don't have to cut away healthy tooth structure just to hold the filling in. So no more creaking noises as the filling is being pushed into the tooth—patients like that.

Composites are also less destructive to the tooth over time. Anything man-made wears at a different rate than the tooth structure, but one of the problems with the silver amalgam fillings is that the material doesn't give as much. When the silver amalgam filling is put in, the patient bites down on some papers to help in adjusting the bite; the filling is shaped so that the bite is hitting on tooth structure and not hammering the filling. Over time, the tooth structure wears and the patient starts hitting on both the filling and the tooth structure. Since the amalgam doesn't give as much, it can become a liability and starts cracking the tooth because it's like a wedge in the center of the tooth.

Still, even the composite resin comes with pros and cons. It wears a little faster than tooth structure, which may cause the filling to leak at some time and have to be replaced. But, so far, we've never seen a composite filling at any time crack a tooth or knock the cusp off a tooth, which is something we see every week with the old amalgams.

ORAL CANCER SCREENING

In the past decade, we've discovered that identifying oral cancer early is key and that since dentists are the ones who are always looking into people's mouths, they're the best ones to do the screening. As a result, oral cancer detection has become a procedure being offered in the dental community.

There are a lot of risk factors involved, particularly for people who smoke. Early detection is important in combating oral cancer. Often, by the time it can be seen by the naked eye, it has already progressed considerably. But we have new tools for early detection, and now oral cancer screening is part of your evaluation during cleaning visits, which occur every six months.

In addition to a visual inspection, we also use the VELscope, which involves shining a light into the mouth and looking through a lens for tissue of a certain color, identifying abnormalities. If a problem is identified, we refer the patient to an oral surgeon for testing or a biopsy. Many patients that we send to the surgeon find there are no real problems. But while we feel we sometimes may be acting a little too cautiously, patients don't seem to mind. They would rather know for sure because if an abnormality is caught early, it's much easier to treat. And without a deeper examination, you can't be sure something isn't wrong.

THE TREATMENT OF PERIODONTAL DISEASE

We specialize in the treatment of periodontal disease. And through this area of our practice, we are truly saving lives. It sounds corny, but it's true; with infections leading to heart problems, it definitely does save lives.

How exactly does gum disease relate to heart problems?

From a simplified standpoint, if you have bacteria in your mouth that stays there and leads to infection, it can get to your heart and cause problems there. When you've got a source of infection in your mouth, deep pockets filled with bacteria develop. If we don't take care of those, they can lead to further problems with the heart or with the brain. Gum disease can also be a sign of other diseases that are not well controlled, such as diabetes.

Gum disease is also the number-one cause of tooth loss and underlying bone loss, which we've already discussed. In short, gum disease leads to the deterioration of the bone, which can eventually lead to tooth loss; if there's not enough bone there, you're going to lose your teeth. Conversely, the loss of a tooth can also lead to deterioration of the underlying bone.

TREATING GUM DISEASE

Our protocol for scaling and root planning to treat gum disease—also known as conventional, nonsurgical periodontal therapy—starts with our highly trained hygienist performing a perio-probing, which measures six sites on each tooth. If the "pocket" of the diseased gum, which is the space between the tooth and the gum, is five millimeters deep or greater, or we can't get into that pocket manually with a toothbrush, then we have to employ a specific type of cleaning—a saline-type procedure using an ultrasonic scaler—to flush out the bacteria in an effort to rid the disease. This can't be done with a regular cleaning.

The ultrasonic scaler actually interrupts that calculus—or tartar—on the tooth; even if we don't get it all off at that point, the scaler kills that calculus, breaking the bond that adheres it to the tooth and causing it to eventually fall off. Even residual calculus is removed at the microscopic level.

Deep pockets—again, five millimeters or greater—are also treated with antibiotics; we use a plastic-tipped, needleless syringe to physically place antibiotics in the pocket. There are various types of antibiotics, including a gel or a powder that must be mixed. While the scaling helps clean the surface, the antibiotic keeps the tooth or teeth bacteria-free for a period of time, allowing for healing and reattachment of the gum tissue to the base of the tooth.

Depending on the number of pockets, we may also do a round of oral antibiotics. For example, if someone comes in with 12 or more pockets, around both arches, top and bottom, we may do a week's worth of oral antibiotics. For ten sites or less, we'll physically place antibiotics in the bottom of the pockets to regain the attachment there so that there won't be pocketing.

We reevaluate the site after a few weeks, and during that time we instruct the patient not to disturb the area; this is one of the few times we tell the patient not to floss or use toothpicks because we don't want them to dislodge the treatment. That doesn't give them a free lifetime pass from flossing; it's just a brief freebie in this particular area while we're getting it to heal. The patient still needs to brush and rinse; we just don't want them in there physically disturbing the treated pocket. The body has to absorb the antibiotic so that it will do its job.

Sometimes we also prescribe Periomed, which is a type of fluoride rinse. This rinse has other ingredients in it, but it's one that we find helps the gum tissue. We use it for gum therapy because it helps with decay, and the fluoride it contains also helps with any sensitivity issues. So we like it best for gum treatment, but it does have other benefits.

The extent of the gingivitis or periodontal disease, along with personal variations in healing time from diabetes, a long list of medications, and other factors determine how long the healing will take. For example, gum issues are a very big problem with diabetic patients; with periodontal disease, their healing time is a little bit longer. Other patients that don't have good home-care habits need to make a concerted effort to reinstate those.

That's why, four to six weeks after the initial treatment, we have patients return to the office so that we can check the probing depths of the pockets again, and as long as we're seeing improvement, we know we're on the right track. If we're not seeing improvement or if we're losing ground, we'll go back into that area again.

If we are seeing healing, then we'll see the patient again in about three months for another cleaning and a reprobe of the pockets to ensure we're seeing improvement. If, at the four-to-six-week point, we've established that everything is progressing, then the restorative and cosmetic procedures can begin.

Gum Disease Is Not Your Fault

Many patients hesitate to address their dental health because there's a certain amount of shame involved.

But some of the factors that cause gum disease are really beyond the patient's control.

For instance, one factor behind gum disease is genetics. We all know that genetic factors like eye color, hair color, and hair patterns are passed along. And sometimes, because of genetics, one person is not as healthy as the next.

Dealing with the problem starts by acknowledging it. Then, you must learn to manage these genetic failings, and you do that by taking whatever precautions or measures are needed.

Beyond genetics, there are other unavoidable factors that make it difficult to battle gum disease.

Age is one such factor. We're hard on our teeth, and by the time we've reached the fifth decade of life or beyond, we've been working our teeth a long time. By then, the amount of pressure that we've put our teeth under and the force that we use with them can create some of these problems.

Many people think that, as long as they stay healthy throughout their lives, their teeth will also remain healthy. That's true to some extent, but as other parts of the body age and become lower functioning, the pH level or salivary flow of the mouth can also change. Some of the chronic conditions of the body that arise over time—high blood pressure or cholesterol, thyroid or heart disease—require medication, which can also cause changes in the mouth, leading to decay and cavity issues.

Sometimes it's simply a matter of life getting in the way. People get busy or have economic hardships, and their dental care lapses. The mouth is really about the only place on the body that someone will allow to bleed on a daily basis without seeking professional help. They'll brush their teeth every morning and spit a small amount of blood when they rinse, but they won't seek help, because nothing hurts. But if someone's eye bled every morning, rest assured, they would seek help.

We also see adults that, for whatever reason, never had proper orthodontic care. Sometimes it's economics, and sometimes it's just a trait throughout the generations that dental care was never a priority. Whatever the reason, their teeth are crooked or misaligned, and it's harder to clean teeth when they're crowded in the mouth.

We want patients to know that we have more advances available today to help correct even lifelong problems.

Digital X-rays

To put it in perspective, you get more exposure to radiation in the summertime outside than you do inside the dental office using digital X-rays.

In digital X-rays, a sensor is used instead of the film that goes in a traditional X-ray machine. One sensor is used to take all of the X-rays. The process still uses radiation, so the X-ray tech has to wear the lead vest, but the X-ray process itself uses 90 percent less radiation.

With digital, we can take a full series of X-rays—18 pictures—and use less radiation than would have been used taking only a couple of bitewings, which were a type of dental X-ray taken with film.

In addition, the images are sharper, and they can be viewed immediately because they display on the computer, which is equipped with software that allows the pictures to be manipulated for clarity. In the past, X-rays were only as good as the person taking the picture, and the film had to be run through chemicals to be developed, which took nearly ten minutes.

Now, even if the first attempt with digital doesn't produce perfect images, the pictures can be retaken immediately because of the low levels of radiation.

With digital X-rays, we see the height of bones, so we can see if we're dealing with bone loss. Or, if the tartar has been on the teeth long enough, we can see that buildup. It's a great diagnostic tool not just for cavities but also for periodontal disease.

The size of the sensor is the same size as the film was in a traditional X-ray, but there's more comfort because it doesn't have the sharp edges.

The digital files are also easy to email to other specialists, such as an oral surgeon or endodontist.

Oral Health 101: The Patient Is an Active Partner

No matter what problems a patient may have when they come in, we're glad they've come, and we're going to address any issues they have and manage them the best we can.

Sometimes we have to prioritize care—maybe the patient has two kids in college, maybe they've got to pay off some debt—and we understand that those issues may come first.

But we try to explain how we're a caring practice and that we will never do dentistry *to* them—we will do dentistry *for* them and *with* them. We want them to fully understand everything that's going on and everything we're going to do. We welcome their questions and input because we're going to do work that's useful and that looks good, and they need to be a part of that.

That's the hallmark of our total transformational model: whether you're having general dentistry work done, correcting a problem to improve your health, or getting one of our cosmetic procedures to enhance your appearance, we want you happy when you walk out the door, and we want you to come back.

After an initial evaluation in our office, a hygienist helps address your specific issues. If you're someone who has not had a regular regimen of home care, chances are you're dealing with some kind of gingivitis or gum problem. For these patients, our hygienist usually talks about the importance of not only brushing but also brushing at least twice a day and for a specific length of time.

Most dental care mistakes can be easily corrected to get your regimen back on track.

Here are some of the essentials you should be doing at home. These can make a big difference in the overall state of your oral health.

1. **Brush at least twice a day**. Whenever possible, children and adults should brush after every meal. But when

brushing that often isn't an option, then children and adults should make sure they're brushing two times every day.

2. **Brush for at least two minutes.** Too often, people just quickly whisk a brush around their mouth. But for brushing to be really effective, it should last at least two minutes. Teaching tots to brush? Tell them to put on a song, and brush while the song is playing.

3. **Use a soft-bristled toothbrush.** A medium- or hard-bristled toothbrush can actually wear out teeth and gums.

4. **Don't apply too much pressure when brushing.** Brushing too hard can cause gums to recede. If you're going through a toothbrush every two months, you're probably applying too much pressure when you're brushing.

5. **Change out your toothbrush.** Toothbrushes need to be changed every three months. If the bristles of a brush are flaring out, it's not working as efficiently as it should. Brushes should also be changed out after a person has been sick with a major illness, such as strep throat.

6. **Use other options for cleaning.** Older adults often don't have sufficient manual dexterity because of arthritis or the effects of aging. So an electric toothbrush such as a Sonicare or a Waterpik is a good option for these individuals. These tools help clean the teeth and remove bacteria under the gums, and they stimulate the gum tissue without

damaging it. You can also use Listerine in the Waterpik to help fight bacteria.

7. **Use mouthwash**. An antimicrobial mouthwash can help keep bacteria at bay. However, some of these contain alcohol, which is not advised for people with dry mouth or chemical dependency issues. There are alcohol-free and prescription rinses available. These are not antimicrobial, but they can help control plaque, gum infection, decay, and sensitivity. Some of these contain stannous fluoride, which is a great fighter of severe periodontal disease when used in conjunction with scaling and root planing in the dentist's office.

8. **Floss daily.** Regular flossing is the first line of defense because cavities typically occur in between teeth. A Waterpik is a good option for people who simply won't floss or don't have the manual dexterity to do so. When flossing, the floss should be wrapped around the tooth like the letter "C," then let go of one end, and pull the floss through.

9. **Use fluoride.** Use of fluoride is important for all ages, not just for children. This is especially true for someone who's had a lot of restorations or gum recession. Use fluoride toothpaste at home, and get fluoride treatments when visiting the dentist.

10. **Get regular cleanings at the dentist.** In general, it's recommended to visit the dentist at least every six months for a regular cleaning and checkup. However, scientific research

has proven that cleanings every three months result in a healthier mouth. The research found that the biofilm—the colonies of bacteria that naturally form in the mouth—begin to gain a foothold at around three months. Disrupting this biofilm at the three-month mark helps reduce damage in the mouth. People with severe and active periodontal disease need to see their dentist more often. The success of treatment for periodontal disease often depends on the homework done by the patient; this also lengthens the time between visits to the dentist for care of the disease.

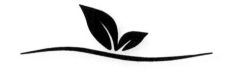

Chapter Three

COSMETIC DENTISTRY: SO MUCH TO SMILE ABOUT

In recent years, patient demand has led to a new focus on cosmetic dentistry. Two generations ago, it was more about function than esthetics; back then, composite resin and tooth color restorations were in their infancy. But whether the popularity has been driven by advertising or the movies, today, people want a brighter smile, and they want their teeth to function well.

When a person does something cosmetic to change their appearance, whether it's dental or something like a new hairstyle or color, they feel better. For some people, a new look is a new beginning or a new phase in their life—maybe they're starting a new job, or they've sent the last child off to college—so they're coming in to get orthodontics, cosmetic dentistry, or Botox.

These days, people want a variety of procedures to enhance the appearance of their smile. For example, we have different types of porcelain, from veneer to all-ceramic crowns, which look good and function well. These and other advances available today are much better than the options we had when we first started practicing.

While oral health provides a foundation for building a beautiful smile, unfortunately not all healthy mouths are as attractive as they could be.

A patient may have no probing depths, healthy gum tissue, and no current decay. They may have some fillings or crowns, but one of those crowns may be a 15-year-old porcelain fused to a metal crown. That porcelain looks very different from the porcelain that we use today. And while they may not have pocketing, they may have some slight rotations in their teeth that make their smile less attractive than it could be.

So some people have a healthy mouth, but their smile is just not as nice as it could be. And studies have found that the smile is a reflection of how a person feels about himself or herself, and that if you're not smiling, you aren't perceived as friendly and warm. The lack of a beautiful smile can have an impact on self-esteem, and it can affect relationships and a person's livelihood.

It's not about vanity. It's just about feeling good about yourself, and everyone deserves that. But sometimes it takes a great smile just to keep you going during the day. The joke around our office is that you can get up every morning and tell the mirror, "Good morning, gorgeous," and that's the only time someone's going to say that to you all day.

WHITENING FOR A BETTER SMILE

One of the first steps in improving your smile is through whitening because it's noninvasive and doesn't change your tooth structure. It allows you to see something of a change, and it opens the door to knowing what it feels like to have a brighter smile. Many patients who have this done start seeing other aspects they might want to change, such as a tooth that's a little bit turned or has a chip.

Patients can go to the store and buy over-the-counter whitening products, but the quality and effectiveness of these products range from very good to very poor.

For example, some of the whitening strips may be good products; the adhesive strip that holds the bleaching agent will bleach whatever surface on the tooth it touches. But the problem is that the tooth is not flat—it's curved, so the strip can miss areas.

There are also rinses available, but they're so diluted that there's just not that much of the lightening ingredient in them. Plus, it's hard to keep rinse on the tooth structure long enough to be of any real benefit.

In the end, if the over-the-counter products really worked, then people wouldn't be coming to us for a better option.

In the office, we put the bleach on the teeth, either with a brush or held against the teeth with a mouthpiece. This allows the bleach to stay on the surface of the teeth longer, or at least for the length of time that it needs to stay, and it gets in between the teeth, covering even the curved part of the tooth surface.

One of the most popular products we offer now is a system that includes a tray containing the whitening bleach along with a session with a special light. We insert the tray into the patient's mouth, and then they sit under the light for 20 minutes.

We then send the patient home with that tray and a bleaching pen with a brush applicator. This allows the patient to apply the bleach directly to the teeth in front of a mirror at home, and then insert the tray to hold the bleach in place. The tray keeps saliva from diluting the bleach, and it keeps the lips from rubbing the bleach off.

It's a much better system than squirting the bleach into the tray, which is how it used to work. The patient would get a syringe and squirt the bleach into the tray, and then put the tray in their mouth. But undoubtedly, they would never get the exact amount of bleach in the tray, and then when it was inserted, the bleach would squeeze out on the gums and just be wasted. The brush applicator allows for better control.

We've had huge success with the new system. People like it because it's easy. They get a good jumpstart in our office—we can usually make the teeth anywhere from three to five shades lighter with the patient sitting under the light with the tray in. Then they do more at home—we've seen bleaching by as much as three shades whiter with the take-home system.

We also do what some call a one-hour power bleaching, where we apply the bleach to the teeth and the patient is under the light for an hour. With this product, we reapply the bleach every 15 minutes to reoxygenate it and make it a little more active. This product requires the patient to sit longer in the chair; they need to be able to sit there and sit still so that the light is hitting the teeth correctly. With this one-hour whitening system, we can get the teeth up to ten shades lighter.

The level of whitening we're able to achieve depends on the type of stains we're dealing with or what made the teeth dark. If food or drink is the cause, that's one thing. But some people have a tetracycline staining caused by medicine, which adds almost a bluish-tan tint to their teeth. This type of stain will not bleach as well, so it's harder for people with tetracycline staining or those on some long-term medicines to get the results they want.

Smoke is a little bit hard also. We get good results with smokers, but there's still the tar, so we get maybe a little darker shade than what's possible with nonsmokers.

The type of whitening we do is really a matter of patient preference. Patients seem to be gravitating toward the 20-minute system because of the cost and the length of time it takes.

We also offer a bleaching-for-life program, which begins with a 20-minute jumpstart bleaching following a cleaning (the best time to bleach is after a cleaning). Then we continue to supply the patient with a take-home brush applicator free of charge as long as they come in for scheduled cleanings.

We find the bleaching-for-life program to be a big motivator; once patients see how good they can look, they keep bleaching on their own, and they keep coming in for appointments.

Some find it fits their lifestyle perfectly to just apply the bleach and insert the tray at the end of the day. For some, it influences a change in lifestyle because the results vary depending on what happens in the mouth throughout the day. For example, if you bleach in the afternoon and then go out for dinner that evening and have red wine, you could actually be staining your teeth even more. The red wine, which is one of the major stain-causing things that a patient can put in the mouth, would soak into the enamel and be able to reach as deep as the bleach had gone. It is best not to put anything in your mouth after bleaching for at least a couple of hours if possible. It is kind of like washing your face with warm water, which opens your pores, and then going out to work in the yard. The pores in your skin would get clogged with dirt. If you bleach, especially right after cleaning, the rods that make up the enamel are open, which allows the bleach in. Once they get coated with saliva and other substances such as food and drink, they're not as open.

We educate patients about how their choices affect the results of their whitening efforts. We're not going to tell you that you can only drink water from here on out, but you should know that coffee, tea, colas, red wine, and smoke are the biggest contributors to staining teeth.

VENEERS AND COMPOSITE BONDING

Veneers and composite bonding are the next steps in the cosmetic continuum.

Composite bonding is a resin that is applied directly to the tooth; it's a direct bonding. The tooth is first prepared with a handpiece; then the etching gel is applied, and the tooth is light cured, shaped, and polished for the look that we want. It has to look and function like a tooth.

Sometimes it's done if someone has a space between teeth; for example, the procedure is performed on two adjacent teeth to close the space between them. We also do bonding out on the edge of the front teeth. It looks good, but the patient has to be careful with it because just the act of eating can chip the restoration; when we eat, we put the front teeth together and they make a shearing action. Hard foods like carrots or apples can be difficult on composites; a fingernail biter can break bonding off very easily.

Veneers are more durable than composites, but they require a little more design, along with laboratory fabrication, and they're more expensive than composites.

Veneers are often referred to as "instant orthodontics" because if a tooth has a little bit of rotation or wear, or it's just crowding a little, a veneer will give an appearance that the arch form is more symmetrical.

The veneer itself is a thin porcelain covering that's designed with the help of our digital imagery. We take an impression of the prepped tooth and send it to the lab; the process is very similar to prepping for a crown. Based on the impression, the lab then makes the veneer out of porcelain. Once the veneer is sent back to us from the lab, it is adhered to the tooth with a type of bonding or cementation.

Before prepping the tooth and taking an impression, we start with X-rays of the tooth to make sure everything's healthy. Then the prepping is done so that we're allowed to get the shape we need while leaving the function of the teeth. The preparation for a veneer is a very conservative prep; we're not taking away a lot of the tooth structure, but we're taking away the amount that's needed to gain the thickness of the porcelain while also taking into account look and strength.

The prep is done with a handpiece, similar to when we're removing a cavity from a tooth. We typically take away a minimal amount of the tooth to prepare the surface for bonding—we round sharp edges and rough the enamel a little so that it bonds a little better

With veneers, we have to look at the entire face—not just the smile—because a veneer has to look symmetrical. We have to go by certain landmarks that are not just in the mouth but also in the face. Some patients have an oval-shaped face, some a square, and some a triangle, so the shape of the teeth has to be considered. We can't put square-shaped veneers on a woman with a nice triangular face; it just won't look right. So we have to look at all of the features of the face.

After the tooth is prepped, we take an impression to send to the lab, where a veneer is made.

Often, we have to fabricate a temporary veneer for the patient while the real veneers are being made. If the tooth is rotated or flared out some, there's more prepping involved. If we have to go through the enamel, we fabricate a temporary so the patient does not experience any sensitivity while the veneer is being made. In a case like that, we make a temporary veneer out of composite.

A standard veneer typically includes six to eight teeth per arch—usually the front eight teeth; this requires a two- or three-week turnaround from the lab.

Most of our veneers are custom veneers. We don't do the snap-on type of veneer. However, we have used a product called Lumineers. Although Lumineers are considered to be "no-prep" veneers, we've never been able to place them on a tooth without some degree of prepping.

One reason we prep the tooth is because we need the enamel a little rougher for the bonding. We also prep to remove sharp edges; a sharp edge underneath porcelain is asking for failure.

Veneers are also custom shaded. If we're doing a complete case of veneers, which usually involves all of the teeth in a patient's smile, most people want them to look completely the same from top to bottom. If we're doing just one or two teeth, which are the hardest matches in the mouth, then we'll have the lab ceramist—the person who's actually going to make those veneers—come in and do the custom shading. The ceramist will do custom shading on the front end and then do a little customization during the cementation phase. That's a benefit of having a lab nearby.

The only pitfall of veneers is that although they look great, their durability is limited. Anything manmade has a certain lifespan and that's it. Some of the earlier porcelains looked great but weren't very durable. Patients used to say, "I can smile with them, but that's it." And that's not really a benefit to the patient, even though some people will put up with anything to look good.

But now the porcelains are so much better. As long as the bite is correct, and there are no other issues, the patient should be able to get 10 or 20 years out of the veneers.

ORTHODONTIA

The main reason for orthodontia is to get the teeth to function correctly—so that there isn't undue wear, periodontal issues aren't created, and there isn't more pressure on one side of the mouth than the other. When the teeth are lined up correctly and function correctly, the by-product is that they look nice.

Orthodontia literally makes the teeth last longer because the bite is more even throughout the arch. It also makes the teeth easier to clean, which helps with the periodontal aspect; teeth that are lined up side by side are easier to floss, easier to maintain, and easier to keep free of food than teeth that overlap.

Like other aspects of dentistry, orthodontia has come a long way. There are just more options today than before.

In the past, orthodontics meant putting a band around every tooth, which meant flaring the teeth out just to get the braces on. The bands were uncomfortable on their own, but then there was also a bracket on each tooth for the wire, so there was a lot more hardware in the mouth. The orthodontic assistant would put in an instrument that the patient had to bite down on to seat the band, but if the patient didn't bite hard, it wouldn't seat. Orthodontic assistants were hated because of that; they were the ones who had to get those bands in, and sometimes the bands would go up under the gum tissue—not a great way to make friends with a 10- or 11-year-old kid.

Today, there may still be bands around some of the molars in the back, but for the most part, brackets are bonded to the teeth, and then the wire runs through the brackets. So it's a kinder procedure that way. There are also different designs of the brackets that hold the wire.

It used to be that the bracket was on the band that was around the tooth—a wire went through the bracket, and then another wire was used to attach that wire. Everything was just packed in the mouth so tight, and the ortho team would have to go in and bend the wire to make it move the teeth. Plus, the wires themselves stuck out so far they'd puff out the patient's lips.

Now, some of the brackets have a door on them. The door pops open and the wire goes in the opening, and then the door closes over the wire to lock it in place. But the wire has a little bit of give within the bracket; it's allowed to move because it's active. It also has memory, meaning if you squeeze it with your fingers to form an arch, it bounces back into shape. And normally, the wires are just changed out.

The old wires would go in and be crimped to make them active. Almost like a barbed wire fence; as the wire sags, the farmer has to crimp the wire to make it tighter. It was the same with orthodontics—the orthodontist had to crimp it to make it tighter.

So again, it's a much kinder ortho. And the results are faster because of it.

INVISALIGN

Invisalign is done with a series of clear aligners or mouthpieces, which are put in and progressively change the teeth.

The orthodontist starts by putting together a treatment plan that includes a computerized, three-dimensional model. The model shows the projected movement of the teeth, the length of time the treatment is going to take, and what's going to be done if the lab makes the aligners as prescribed. The aligners are of clear, BPA-free plastic that is practically invisible on the teeth.

Impressions made of the patient's mouth are used to create the entire series of aligners. Aligners are changed out generally every two weeks. But the progression of aligners can be altered if at some point in the treatment it's determined that things aren't going as originally planned. If a change is needed, an entire new set of aligners will be made from that point forward, using new impressions.

The aligners can be removed for eating, which means that, unlike traditional braces, patients aren't restricted from enjoying foods like popcorn, nuts, or any sticky foods. Invisalign also makes it easier to clean the teeth. And when we change out the patient's aligners, we tell patients to make the switch at night before they go to bed because that's when that aligner is the most snug, helping to reduce the patient having to deal with discomfort and soreness. On the whole, patients report that the Invisalign system is less difficult to deal with than the wire system; the first aligner is reportedly the most uncomfortable, but subsequent aligners tend to be far less so.

The number of aligners really depends on the mouth. An advanced case may go through 20–30 aligners; another case may only need 16 on the top and 6 on the bottom.

The Invisalign system doesn't necessarily move the teeth faster than the old methods, and it costs about the same. The main benefit is that the patient is not wearing the bands and brackets, and they're able to eat whatever they want.

Although we don't advise this, the truth is, Invisalign gives the patient more control, so some patients take advantage of the flexibility and don't wear the aligners as much as they should. But the aligners have built-in indicators that let us know whether or not they are being worn enough.

www.invisalign.com

The Importance of a Balanced Bite

The temporomandibular joint, or TMJ, is the ball-and-socket jaw joint that allows a person to open and close and actually move the lower jaw from side to side. It involves bone, cartilage, blood vessels, nerves, and muscle.

Disorders of the TMJ—the breakdown of the joint resulting in pain, popping, and clicking—is known as TMD, or temporomandibular disorder. TMD occurs as a result of the wear and tear on the joint itself. We've seen X-rays of patients where the ball part of the joint is worn flat; it's similar to a worn-out hip joint. We can almost guarantee when we look in the mouth that we're going to see a certain wear pattern if the ball and socket is worn on one side more than the other.

Ideally, when the TMJ and surrounding muscles are functioning properly and all the teeth are aligned and in place, your bite is in balance.

But sometimes people get tense and clench those muscles, get hit while playing sports, or strain the muscles by constantly gritting their teeth, and their bite gets thrown out of balance.

There's cartilage between the two bones of the joint— the ball and the socket—that acts as a cushion. If you've been around someone whose jaw pops when they eat or when they yawn, that's the cartilage being pinched by the bone. It's popping either forward or back, behind that ball and socket. That's where it keeps pinching, and it keeps damaging the cartilage; that's when you start getting into chronic problems with the jawbone.

In addition to the noise, if the joint is not working properly, then the teeth don't come together correctly. The patient can start getting soreness of teeth because one site may be hitting harder than the other when the patient chews. Sometimes, TMD results in cracked or chipped teeth or broken restorations. If the teeth get worn down, you can also get a prematurely aged appearance; the nose starts getting close to the chin just like the caricature of a Halloween witch.

The jaw pain can also manifest as headaches and pain all the way down into the neck and shoulders because the muscles that go down there greatly affect the jaw and the side of the head.

Some patients may appear to be relaxed and laid back when we first meet them. If we watch them talk and chew and watch the facial muscles, we can tell the people who are used to clenching or grinding because the muscle that runs up the side of the head—called the masseter—bulges out. If we look in the mouth we can see the wear on the teeth and feel the tightness of the muscle.

We're very fortunate in our office to have two assistants who are also massage therapists. They have brought a lot to the table for our patients with TMJ problems. Both have been able to give relief to patients that deal with TMD and the uncomfortable symptoms that comes with it.

In addition to visual cues, we also talk to patients to find out where they are in life. It's not unusual to find people in college who have never been grinders or clenchers in their life but who come home on Christmas break and complain of being tired and having a sore mouth and headaches. We find that they're big-time clenching. They just finished finals, or they just came through a tough science class that kicked their tail for the last four months. TMD happens when problems arise in a person's life.

Treating TMD ranges from applying heat to the muscle, to using a mouthpiece or a bite guard, or to administering Botox. A lot of clenchers use a habit appliance—a night guard—which does not necessarily stop them from the act of closing down and trying to apply pressure. But if a mouth guard is in between the teeth, it keeps the upper teeth off the lower teeth; it does not allow the mouth to close all the way. The muscles may still be closing, but they can't contract all the way and apply full pressure, thereby damaging the teeth.

Some people say the smell of lavender helps them. Some of our patients say they use a lavender candle at night, or they take a hot bath, or they get a washcloth and put it in the hottest water they can stand and then place it on their jaw joint before they go to bed.

If a patient has lived with pain for years and now has an unbalanced bite, they might need more aggressive treatment. That may involve restoration, because often the tooth structure is already worn down so much that the patient is literally over-closing. Sometimes it's a full-mouth restoration with crowns and bridges, and sometimes it's creating a more definitive stop with their back teeth.

Orthodontics, or moving the teeth, is an excellent way to treat TMD because that's treating the entire arch, and it's not pressing away tooth structure. Also, by aligning the teeth up and evening out the bite, we're preventing problems down the road.

Botox is another option because it relaxes the muscles for longer periods of time. Botox binds to the muscle for about three months and doesn't allow the muscle to contract. It doesn't paralyze the muscle; its job is to relax the muscle to allow better function—not to take function away.

Botox is often considered a frontline treatment to TMJ problems and headache pain. If the pain is created by a muscle, Botox may treat the problem by relaxing that muscle. Botox will not, however, heal a damaged bone or the cartilage.

Botox also provides a diagnostic advantage: if we put it in and there's no relief, then we know the muscle is not the problem. Then the Botox clears from the body in 90 days. Botox can also be used as a pain-easing strategy before doing orthodontia; once the pain is gone, we explain that properly aligning the teeth can also give the patient the same feeling and the same relief.

The Mouth's pH Balance

Many patients experience the condition xerostomia, commonly known as dry mouth.

Dry mouth changes the pH balance in the mouth. Saliva acts as a buffer to neutralize acids in the mouth, so once it's gone, the mouth is very prone to decay and sensitivity. Dry mouth is a very uncomfortable condition: the cheeks and tongue can stick to the teeth, and it's very difficult to swallow. Dry mouth can even contribute to bad breath.

Dry mouth is typically caused by any number of commonly used medications and medical conditions. Blood pressure and antianxiety medicines are two of the most common culprits of dry mouth, but oncology patients also deal with dry mouth because treatments change the mouth's pH.

People who experience dry mouth often believe it's just a condition they have to live with. Drinking or sipping water, chewing gum, or consuming mints—ideally with an artificial sweetener such as xylitol—can help stimulate salivary flow.

There are also lubricating rinses and other options available to combat dry mouth and its side effects. These include over-the-counter rinses and gels. Some of the rinses contain enzymes that encourage salivary flow to help reduce dry mouth. The gel form is typically for rubbing on the different surfaces inside the mouth purely for comfort.

Cosmetic Dentistry: Do Your Homework

For real success after a cosmetic procedure, it's important for patients to do their homework to help maintain and optimize results.

For starters, it's important to keep up with oral hygiene. Be sure to follow a regular regimen of brushing and flossing to keep teeth healthy and strong.

If you've had professional whitening done, follow up the in-office procedure with the tray and bleaching pen supplied by the dentist. The new brush applicator system makes application of the bleach an easy-to-perform component in maintaining beautiful, white teeth.

For the best results, bleach right after brushing, and reduce consumption of staining foods and drinks such as coffee, tea, colas, red wine, and spaghetti sauce.

Taking care about what you eat is also important if you have veneers or composites. Crunchy or sticky foods— candied apples, popcorn balls, etc.—can really damage these types of dental work.

And with orthodontia, it's important to continue to regularly wear the retainer or final aligner to help keep newly aligned teeth in place. Teeth have memory and will try to shift back to their original positions if a nightly retainer isn't worn. The Invisalign system comes with a Vivera retainer, which is made of a sturdier material that is designed to be worn at night for at least the first year after treatment.

Chapter Four

RESTORATIVE DENTISTRY: GETTING THE SMILE YOU ALWAYS DESERVED

While preserving your natural teeth is the top goal of modern dentistry, sometimes teeth simply cannot be saved.

First, we'll sketch out a few reasons why we lose teeth, but note that such circumstances needn't keep you from smiling, thanks to a range of incredibly durable—and incredibly good-looking—restoration options.

We've already touched on some of the reasons people lose teeth. Sometimes life gets in the way and affects the health of the mouth. Genetic reasons can cause tooth loss; some people are just not as healthy as others. And accidents happen—not only automobile accidents but also accidents around the home, such as when a toddler cracks a parent's tooth by head-butting him in the mouth while the parent is picking them up.

Just because you can't save a natural tooth doesn't mean you can't have a smile that you feel good about.

We have a number of patients who can attest to that.

For example, a local high school basketball coach thanked us for making him look good—ultimately because of how we treated one of his star players.

Eight years prior, the student had braces on his teeth. During a game, he was hit so hard that one of his teeth was knocked completely out of its socket. The only thing holding the tooth in was the bracket of the orthodontics.

We replanted the tooth and made it stable. The student ended up having a root canal and had to have the tooth restored, but he was able to keep the tooth. Today, he is scoring 30 or 40 points a night in games. The coach said he appreciated the care we provided because the student could have gone anywhere to high school but chose to stay here because of the care he receives and the people in the area.

That's what restorative dentistry is all about: saving the natural tooth. And again, today there is a range of incredibly durable, incredibly good-looking restoration options. The materials are better, and the techniques have improved greatly, not only for restoring the teeth that we keep but also for restoring missing teeth or the spaces where teeth are missing.

Restoration of a tooth entails restoring the natural, existing tooth. The tooth needs restoring if it has a cavity, which is decay, or if it's worn down, chipped, or cracked, or if it gets abscessed from clenching or grinding. The tooth is staying intact; it's just being restored.

When circumstances are such that the natural tooth can't be restored, then we have durable options. We restore teeth that are missing—whatever the reason for the loss—to preserve the patient's oral health and overall health. Restorations for missing teeth are done because we're trying to fill that void with something to maintain the integrity of the arch, whether it's the top or the bottom arch. Arch integrity is important because normally everyone has two molars per side of that arch, and if one is lost, then that's half of the surface area of the compression forces used to chew our food.

Some people think that if the tooth that's gone is in the very back, then they won't miss it. But if it's the next-to-the-last tooth, then not only have you lost that tooth, but if you don't restore that space—if you don't put something back in—the tooth behind it is going to shift forward. And it won't move forward as if sliding a chess piece across the board; instead, it *tilts* forward. Also, the tooth above it is going to start to drop down. That's what we mean by maintaining the integrity of the arch.

We also restore missing teeth to maintain the integrity of the face. As we mentioned before, when teeth are gone, the facial muscles and the anatomy of the face change over time, and the face tends to sink in.

Restoration helps you avoid the consequences we discussed more extensively in the previous chapter.

FILLINGS

A restoration that is a filling is considered a direct restoration, meaning that the cavity or the decay is removed from the tooth. That's what we use the handpiece for. Then, the restoration, or the filling, is placed directly in the tooth. As we discussed earlier, to do a filling there has to be enough tooth structure to support it; usually, you need more tooth structure than the size of the filling.

The good thing about direct restorations is that the materials are so much better today—both because of natural tooth color and because the materials bond directly to the tooth itself rather than being held in with mechanical retention, which is the case with silver amalgam fillings. With amalgam, even after the decay is removed from the tooth, we have to go in and remove healthy tooth structure just to create undercuts to lock it in. This is one of the main reasons we no longer use amalgam fillings in our practice.

With composite materials, once the decay is removed we don't have to remove any more tooth structure; the material bonds directly to the tooth.

There are different types of composites available today. Most of them are hybrid and made to last longer. Viewed under a microscope, a hybrid composite is composed of large particles for strength along with smaller particles in between, enabling it to be polished so that it will look good and shine. Under magnification, the hybrid composite looks similar to a glass vase that you fill with rocks but then add pebbles. If you shake the vase, the pebbles settle in between the rocks. If you put sand in the vase, it fills even more of the spaces. That's what the newer composites are like: they have all different sizes of molecules for strength and wearability but also for polishability so that they look nice.

The original composites had only larger particles because it was thought that would make them strong enough to stand up to wear. The large particles didn't wear as fast, but once the wear started, they began to leak immediately all the way through. Those early composites had definite advantages as far as preserving the tooth structure and certainly had aesthetic advantages over the amalgams. They weren't necessarily more durable; they were mostly made to be placed in the front of the mouth so that the darker fillings didn't show. The first composites were not recommended for the back teeth.

But new technologies make composites suitable for all teeth. Plus, installation is now much easier, for both the practitioner and the patient.

There is wide concern over mercury in the old silver amalgam fillings. When our dad was in practice, mixing up an amalgam meant adding a couple of drops of mercury to some pellets in a capsule that went into a machine that shook it all up. When it came out, it would be in a state where it could be shaped until it hardened. The mercury's purpose was to make the filling workable for that brief period of time.

But if you had leftover mercury that you didn't want to use anymore, you couldn't dispose of it. The only legal place you can dispose of it is in the patient's mouth, and there's something very backward about that.

By itself, mercury is a toxic substance, and there are studies that show that over time, chewing wears the amalgam down, and that can release vapors. Other studies also show that removing an old filling can release vapors that are toxic to the patient, the dentist, and the dental assistant in the room. Still, we remove amalgam fillings all the time for patients who request that, particularly if the filling is not doing what it was supposed to do—keeping the tooth sealed. Some patients request that we replace the amalgam with composite for health reasons—others want it done for cosmetic reasons. Eventually, because of use and wear, any filling will have to be replaced.

On a graph of toxins, mercury appears to be a very hazardous substance. But in the big scope of things, it's actually very low. For us, it's a hazard of our profession, but so is working with some of the other instruments. Some of our handpieces, for instance, operate with a very high-pitched noise, and we handle those eight hours a day. Over time, that can really damage the hearing.

In the end, mercury is still considered safe to put in the mouth by the American Dental Association and the US government.

We haven't used mercury in nearly two decades—partly because of the concerns with it but more so just because there are better materials available. And why wouldn't we want to use better materials?

Many dentists still use amalgam because that's what insurance companies pay for; composites are typically covered only up to the amount that amalgam costs; the rest is out of pocket for the patient, which, for them, can be significant and cost prohibitive. In our office, insurance typically covers about half the cost of a composite filling.

One factor to consider when looking at amalgam versus composite is longevity.

The size of the filling determines its longevity—the larger the filling, the shorter its lifespan. When the filling is put in, it is shaped up and it has to be supported by tooth structure. The wider that filling gets and the deeper it gets into that tooth structure determines how long it will last for the patient, so it doesn't take long for that tooth structure to wear again before that filling's going to leak. This is true for any direct filling material.

With amalgam, the metal and the tooth don't wear at the same rate, as we discussed in chapter two. Once the tooth structure wears down and the bite starts hitting both tooth and filling, the metal doesn't give as much. And if the filling is larger, it's easy for that filling to act like a wedge and crack a tooth.

It's very similar to splitting a log; when you put a wedge in the log and then hit it with the back of the axe, it splits the log. That's what an amalgam can do to a tooth over time.

Amalgam requires more of the tooth to be removed, thereby sacrificing longevity. These may be factors to weigh when deciding between amalgam and composite.

Sometimes composites need to be replaced, especially with the pressure that they are under in the mouth. But sometimes we don't have to put in a full replacement because two composites can be bonded together. For example, sometimes we'll see a little decay starting to form in the groove that runs in between two composite fillings in the tooth, and it'll start breaking down tooth structure there. If we catch it early enough, we can just remove that unhealthy tooth structure and bond it there—keeping the rest of the filling as long as it's not leaking or creating damage.

CROWNS

The challenge with both amalgam and composite fillings is that, once the filling gets too large, it becomes weaker because we have to remove too much of the tooth to put the filling in. That's usually when we have to go from doing a filling to doing something like a crown, which some people refer to as a cap.

A crown is considered an indirect restoration because the tooth is prepped, an impression is made, and the impression is sent to the lab. Instead of placing the restoration directly in the tooth inside the mouth, as in a filling, a crown is made outside the mouth to fit the model made from the impression, and then it is cemented in.

Crowns are used in cases where decay is so extensive that a filling isn't a good option or an option at all. A crown is used when the damage to a tooth is getting too large for just a filling. In a tooth that has a filling, biting down sends a force either through that filling or onto the cusps of the teeth. In contrast, a crown covers the entire tooth. When there's a crown covering the tooth, biting down distributes force over the entire tooth.

There is another indirect restoration that some people call the three-quarter, or partial crown, or an onlay. The impression is still taken, and the restoration is made outside the mouth, and the onlay is bonded or cemented on, but it only covers one or two cusps instead of all four.

Sometimes a crown is used to get the tooth back to a better function, not just to replace missing tooth structure because of decay. Crowns are used on a tooth that is rotated or shifted a little and when the patient does not want to go through orthodontics. We can prep a tooth so that when the crown is put on, it'll make the tooth look like it is straight.

Crowns are a good solution for teeth that are worn down. As teeth wear down, we lose what is called vertical dimension. This basically means that our nose starts getting closer to our chin, which ages us greatly, but it also puts a lot more pressure on the jaw joint. By restoring the teeth with the crowns, especially teeth that oppose each other or that chew with each other, we create those natural stops with the crowns, which prevent wear.

A crown is also used to protect a tooth that has undergone a root canal. A root canal removes the nerve that runs through the center of the tooth; to take the nerve out, the center of the tooth structure—the inside core—has to be removed. We fill the core with composite or a post made of carbon fiber, nickel titanium, or other material, and then we put the crown over the tooth to help protect when the patient bites down. Again, this distributes force over that entire tooth.

We always have to prep the tooth that is going to get the crown. To prep the tooth, we have to remove some of the structure to allow for the thickness of the material to be added.

Once the tooth is prepped, we have to make sure it's dry. The impression material comes in a double-barrel cartridge that looks like a glorified caulk gun. The material comes in heavy body and light body, the latter of which flows easier. We flow some of the material around the tooth and put some in an impression tray. Once we have the material around the tooth, we insert the filled impression tray in the patient's mouth and press it to the tooth so that we get a nice impression of not only that tooth but also the teeth around it. That gives the lab a model of the mouth exactly the way it was when we had it prepped.

Then we make an impression of the opposing arch, which are the other teeth that chew in this area, so that the lab has a model of exactly how those teeth go together and how they function. It helps the lab fabricate the crown to properly fit in the patient's mouth.

The crown itself is made of a choice of materials: all ceramic, all metal, or mostly gold. There are also porcelain-fused-to-metal crowns where the understructure is metal but porcelain is put on top; the porcelain exterior is the only part visible on these crowns.

Another material that's relatively new to the market is the BruxZir Solid Zirconia crown, which looks like a real tooth but is very hard and very strong.

Most patients don't really care what kind of material we use for the crown: they just want it to fit, feel good, and look good.

Although gold crowns are rare in our office, they offer several benefits that often justify the price a patient may pay. With gold, we don't have to prep away as much tooth structure, and gold is very biocompatible in the mouth—the body responds to gold very well. There is also a gold version with an onlay.

The cost of each of the different crowns varies, and the price of gold affects the cost of a gold crown.

We usually suggest what we think is best for the patient based on durability, esthetics, and other considerations.

For example, if someone wants to replace the front six teeth because they don't like the way their smile is, or they don't like the crack in their teeth or the staining, we'll use a certain type of porcelain in the front because it looks better and it polishes better. Selection may depend on the patient's bite; typically the forces involved are a lot lighter in the front teeth—not as heavy as in the molar area.

Once we fit the patient with a temporary crown, it takes about two to three weeks to get the permanent crown back from the lab. That temporary crown is shaped and polished to fit the prepped tooth; it's fabricated to be the exact size and shape that the tooth was before we even touched it. We use composite to create the temporary crown, and we adhere it with temporary cement. When we need to remove it, we are able to hold onto it with a pair of hemostats, squeeze it a little, and it'll flex just enough to break the seal of the temporary cement and come off very easily. We tell patients to avoid foods that are sticky or crunchy while they're wearing the temporary crown so that they don't dislodge it.

When we seat the crown, we do color shading on it. Our systems are very good and allow us to match to the surrounding teeth. This is especially important with crowns on the front teeth; with these teeth, the lab tech comes to our office and makes the final touch-ups before we cement the crowns in. It takes an extra 20 minutes or so to get the shading just right, but it's well worth it to have teeth that match and look like natural teeth.

We also make sure the crown is a good fit before we cement it in; it needs to function just like the tooth did.

Unfortunately, we've had to remove a few teeth that should have been crowned but weren't. For example, we've extracted teeth that had root canals that went awry because the tooth wasn't protected by a crown. If the tooth isn't restored with a crown, it just shortens the life of the tooth. Without its nerve and inner core, the tooth is not going to have a blood supply or the nutrients running into the inside of the tooth. This makes it brittle over time.

The handpieces we use today are so much better and more efficient than what our father used, so patients are not in the chair as long, and therefore, prep time is greatly shortened.

It's the same with the impression material. We can get impression material that has to stay in the mouth up to maybe three minutes, whereas what we used in dental school or what our dad used in the practice had to stay in the mouth eight minutes. That's a long time.

Today's impression materials also give far superior results. They capture so much more of the landscape—not just the prepped tooth but also the gum tissue around it, which is very important because that also dictates some of the shape of the crown and how the tooth emerges out of the gum tissue. This gives us a better result from the lab.

Since the lab doesn't have the patient, the mouth, the face, or the smile to work with, we try to give it as much information as possible. If we're doing crowns for the front, we also send photos of the face so that the lab techs can see the smile—where the lip goes, how the corners of the mouth react, and so on.

In summary, today we can get much better longevity with these types of restorations because of both better techniques and better materials. It's not just about treating the tooth, however. Today we're really concerned about making sure everything is healthy. If other areas around the tooth aren't whole and aren't healthy, then that crown may not be able to withstand all the pressure put on it. For instance, if the tooth beside it isn't healthy, it could shorten the lifespan of its neighboring tooth. That can still happen today, which is why we try to get the entire mouth healthy and not just on a tooth-by-tooth basis.

Getting to know the patient makes a big difference as well. If we know a patient is under a lot of stress at work, they may break a crown more easily than someone who isn't under that kind of pressure. So the materials make a huge difference, but getting to know our patients makes a significant difference as well.

That's why, for some patients that we know are clenchers or grinders, we'll suggest a mouth guard when they sleep to help protect their investment. Again, we're not just treating the tooth—we're treating the patient and figuring out what's going to give them something that lasts a long time but also functions well for us.

BRIDGES

A bridge actually "bridges" a space or a gap where a tooth is missing, where the entire tooth had to be removed.

If a tooth is gone and there is a tooth on either side of the space— one in front and one behind—we can do a bridge.

Generally, with a bridge, the teeth on either side of the space are prepped just like for a crown, and then a bridge is made to rest on the two prepped teeth, with a connecting tooth in between. It looks like three teeth, but it's cemented to the two adjacent teeth, which are the pillars of the bridge.

A bridge can't go around the arch of the mouth and just rest on two teeth—for example, one molar on each side. There must be multiple pillars, or teeth, to rest on. And the longer the bridge gets, the more stress or strain that's put on it.

Depending on where the bridge is in the mouth, it may rest on two or more teeth. For example, if a person gets one of the front four teeth on the lower level knocked out, we might do a bridge that rests on two teeth on one side of the space for strength because those teeth are so small.

There are bridges that fill a single-tooth space and some that fill a space of more than one tooth. Trying to bridge a gap of more than two or three missing teeth is really pushing the limits. Beyond that distance, as far as the space is concerned, it's best to start looking at a removable partial denture or implants.

Bridges are pretty much made in the same manner and from the same material as crowns. Porcelain alone is not good for longer spans, as it will break under too much pressure; it's best to use porcelain-fused metal to get the support needed.

We prep the pillar teeth and take an impression of them plus the areas where the two teeth are missing. Then the teeth of the bridge are designed to fit that space.

We shape the teeth in the bridge to make the bite function properly, and then we shape so that the teeth look nice—and so that they look like individual teeth even though they're connected together. So, again, with the bridge, we can give someone a natural-looking, esthetically pleasing result.

DENTURES

There are basically two types of dentures: partial and full.

A full denture replaces all of the teeth in either the upper arch or the lower arch. That would be either a complete upper denture or a complete lower denture.

We advise patients to take the complete denture if the teeth just cannot be saved—the teeth can't be restored, there is too much decay, there is periodontal disease, and the patient has recurring infections. Sometimes when the teeth are in bad shape, it's a health issue, and the patient retaining their own teeth when they're unhealthy is making matters worse. Usually the patient feels better once the teeth are removed even if they never wear the dentures.

A partial denture is removable, just like a complete denture, but it only replaces teeth that are missing. The partial rests on gum tissue where the teeth are missing and on the existing teeth in the arch.

A partial denture is a good option where there are too many teeth missing and a bridge is not an option because the space is too large.

The partial can fill in not just larger spaces but also multiple spaces. For example, if the patient has a space on the left side of the mouth on the top and then also on the right side on the top, one partial will fill both those spaces.

So it's an economical option to a bridge, or it's an option when there are too many restorations for a bridge to accommodate.

It's the same thing if a person is missing one premolar on each side of one of their arches in the mouth. If the patient has a space on the left and the right, it could be restored either with two three-unit bridges or one partial denture.

We also have some patients who have a space on each side and want to do bridges but just can't afford them right now, so they'll do a partial just to hold everything in place. The partial still functions; it keeps the teeth from shifting by basically keeping the spaces as they are until the patient can afford to do the bridges. When the patient is able to do one bridge, the partial is altered so that they can still wear it and hold the space on the other side. It's used transitionally until the patient can have the bridge work done.

Our office works with the snap-in type of dentures, which affix to implants in the gums. We maintain the snap-in type because they are equipped with an O-ring, a gasket of sorts, which helps the denture firmly attach to the implant. Because the pH of the mouth is usually acidic, those gaskets have to be replaced periodically to help the dentures stay in place.

We also offer removable dentures, which are held in place by the landscape of the mouth. These are designed to fit the contour of the gum tissue. The challenge with these is that the longer the patient goes without teeth or has teeth that are missing, the more the bone resorbs and the gums recede. The height of the bone changes, so the amount of retention changes, requiring some patients to use over-the-counter adhesives. That's often when patients decide to go with implants.

Some patients prefer to stay with the removable dentures and just have them realigned, refitted, or in some cases, remade. The frequency of this depends on the patient and is sometimes determined by the health of the individual.

On the plus side, removable dentures can help improve the health of a patient's mouth and are a good option for people who cannot afford a full set of implants. But by the time a patient gets to this point, we've really run out of options for saving teeth. There's no reversing out of a complete denture. That's why we try to focus on staying healthy and keeping as many teeth as we can.

Whatever type of restoration we offer, we want to be sure we give the patient realistic expectations. If we're making a denture for a 75-year-old, the patient is not going to have the mouth they had at 18.

The dentures are made of acrylic, and esthetically, some considerations have a lot to do with the patient's gender and age and the shape of his or her face. For example, certain teeth have a kinder shape, which looks better in a female mouth. Also, the color of the gum tissue on the dentures is very different from patient to patient.

With dentures, we take a full impression of the mouth and send it along with photographs to the lab. Rather than just sending an impression—which only gives the lab the impression and the shape of the arch—we also add photos to show the shape of the face and the patient's ethnicity.

Sometimes a patient comes in after wearing a denture for decades, and they'll just want another that fits and feels the same. For these patients, we send an impression of the denture to the lab to have the denture remade. We can also create new impressions of a patient's mouth to give them a better fitting or functioning set of dentures. With both of these scenarios, we also send photos to the lab to allow the techs to see the shape of the face and the size of the lips because we want a certain amount of tooth structure to show in the teeth.

A lot of what we want showing has to do with the age of the patient. When we're younger, we show more of our upper teeth when we talk. As we age, we show more of our lower teeth. So if a patient comes in and tells us their teeth are making them look old, we may have to instruct the lab that we want to show more of the upper teeth because that gives a more youthful look.

IMPLANTS

The implant is a restoration that goes in the space where a tooth is missing without altering the tooth on either side of the space. It doesn't change anything else in the mouth other than where it's going in. Our office restores implants that have been surgically placed by specialists, such as a periodontist or oral surgeon.

A fixed implant is composed of three components: one part—the anchor—is surgically implanted into the bone; the next—the abutment—is fitted and tightened into the anchor with a screw; and the last—the crown—is the actual restoration that is seen in the mouth.

The anchor is made of surgical-grade metal, typically titanium. The abutment screws into the implant (anchor) that's in the bone; a portion of the abutment stays outside the bone and gum tissue, and after it is prepped or fabricated, forms the core for the crown. The crown, or in some cases, a bridge that rests on two different implants, is cemented onto the abutment. The crown is the same as one made for an intact tooth: same material, same procedures. So this is an implant that is restored with a fixed crown or a fixed bridge that cements in and stays in.

There are also implants that go into the bone and that a denture fits onto, but while the implants are fixed, the denture is removable— the patient can insert and remove the denture.

The technology for the first dental implants was developed in the early 1950s by a Swedish scientist. The first true dental implant was put in place in 1965 and still functioned well 40 years later.

Modern dental implants have been around for decades, but they've evolved considerably. Early implants were much larger and consequently needed a considerable amount of supporting bone, which eliminated many candidates. As previously mentioned, once a tooth is missing, the bone starts to resorb. Without enough bone, the dental professional drilling the pilot hole for the anchor risks drilling through the side of the bone, which is an immediate failure.

Some earlier versions of implants involved drilling a trough, of sorts, into the bone, when compared to the cylinders that are drilled in today. Back then, those troughs were state of the art, but today they seem archaic. It just doesn't take that much bone with today's implants. It's sort of like putting up an eight-by-eight inch post at the end of your driveway for your mailbox, when a four-by-four inch post does fine.

In addition to needing less space, implant materials have been fine-tuned over time. Today, they are much stronger. The screws are about the size of eyeglass screws, yet they hold like a surgical pin for a bone break or fracture.

The advantages of implants over restorations include the fact that no other teeth in the mouth have to be altered, whereas with a bridge, a tooth on each side of the space has to be prepped. That prepping requires structure of those adjacent teeth to be removed to cement the bridge on. Often, those adjacent teeth need restoring anyway. But if there's no decay, then instead of taking the enamel off those teeth and prepping them for a conventional bridge, we can save them if we use an implant. We can leave those adjacent teeth just like they are and restore the space.

Another benefit is that implants never decay. There's no cavity, because there's no tooth structure. It still has to be maintained; the bone and gum tissue still have to be cleaned and kept healthy just as if a tooth were there. But titanium doesn't decay.

Although implants can withstand natural forces—the pressure of the bite—they are stationary. A tooth will move; a tooth is dynamic. An implant doesn't move; it doesn't have a ligament around it like the root of a tooth, so it has no give to it. Over time, as we use our teeth, the tooth structure wears down. A restored implant doesn't wear at the same rate, so we have to go in there and lightly adjust or modify it to keep it biting equally with the rest of the teeth that are changing because of wear. And given enough pressure, enough force—for example, from clenching and grinding—a restoration can break.

That's why dentists want to see patients on a regular basis for maintenance. It's not just for cleaning the teeth; it's so we can take a look around and make sure everything is holding up and doing what it's supposed to do.

Again, anything man-made—whether it's an appliance in the kitchen or a restored tooth in the mouth—has a certain lifespan. And as brutal as we are to our teeth and our restorations, some go away sooner than others.

It really depends on the bite. That's why the bite needs to be even, why teeth need to be in alignment, and why restorations need to be formed and shaped so that everything functions as evenly as possible. But it's an ongoing process.

When we identify a candidate in need of a restoration, we begin by giving them options. We tell them about bridges or implants, whichever is most appropriate, and then also give them the option of doing nothing. Usually choosing to do nothing is not a good option, but it still exists.

If the best option is an implant, and the patient agrees, then we refer them to the periodontist or oral surgeon for an implant consultation. The consultation does not obligate the patient to any treatment but just gives them more information on the implants and the process of doing the procedure.

Once an implant is placed, there's a minimum waiting time of six months before it is restored. If it's a tooth in the front, we have to make arrangements to have something on a temporary basis put in that space. Usually it is something removable that the patient takes in and out. It's not ideal in a lot of circumstances, but it's better than walking around with a hole in your smile. That temporary partial is sometimes called a "flipper." It's not a crown, because there's nothing to anchor to, and it's not something the patient can put a lot of pressure on.

Any tooth in the mouth is a candidate for an implant, as long as there is enough bone to support it. Of course, cost can be a factor, as it is with any dental procedure, whether it's an implant or a fluoride treatment. We tell patients our cost, but we aren't able to quote the specialist's fee. A lot of that depends on the condition of the tooth. For example, if the tooth is broken off right at the gumline where it can't be seen in the mouth but the root is still there, the specialists usually want to take the root out themselves and put something in to help preserve bone so that there will be more bone to put an implant in.

There's also better preservation of bone with implants. That helps everyone because once a tooth is removed and the bone starts to resorb, it doesn't just resorb from the top down—it also resorbs from the sides, which not only takes away bone but affects facial features, too.

On occasion, on a front tooth, if the root is straight and very similar in size to the implant, the tooth can be removed and the implant placed so that the bone then heals to the implant as it's healing from the extraction. We more often see the bone being allowed to heal and then going back later and putting the implant in the bone rather than in the actual socket. But it can be done the either way.

Usually these procedures are done under local anesthesia—the same as if it were a crown or other restoration procedure. With difficult cases, and depending on the scheduling, sometimes we'll go to the specialist's office when the implant is being done. It's not required, but it can help us understand the details of a challenging situation—for example, if an implant of a front tooth has to go in at a slight angle to match the angle and the shape of the tooth that was in the space.

We also work with oral surgeons who do implants if the patient has a prior relationship with that professional. But for referrals, we typically go with a periodontist because their responsibility is the care of the entire foundation of the mouth, which is bone and gum tissue. It's not just placing an implant in bone; the tissue around it also has to stay healthy, so the periodontist sees the patient on a maintenance basis, too.

In addition to restorative procedures on new implants, we see patients when there's a problem with an implant—for example, if a crown breaks, the implant starts to loosen, or gum issues such as resorption develop.

We start by looking for the root of the cause; most of the time, the issue involves something more systemic than just the tooth itself. Often it involves other health issues, such as a medicine the patient is on, or just an overall lack of care because something is going on in the patient's life that is distracting them from their oral health. If it's one of these problems, then the patient may have to see the periodontist or his physician to begin care.

If, as we mentioned earlier, the problem is caused by the wearing down of surrounding teeth, then we're able to lightly adjust the crown so that the bite is more even. Or sometimes it involves restoring the surrounding teeth with similar materials so that there's more even wear throughout the entire arch, not just in one area—we'll put a restoration on the surrounding teeth and then shape and polish them up to get the correct contour. We want to restore the surface of the teeth and the bite so that they are more even and can withstand the pressure.

If the problem is a worn edge that's developed from too much force, such as grinding or clenching, then we can adjust the bite with a handpiece with a very fine polishing diamond—more of a polishing surface than anything. It's like filing a fingernail; we just graze across the tooth in a certain area to make it hit on the mouth as evenly as the other side.

We also redo the restoration (crown) on implants for esthetic reasons. For example, we don't gain more gum tissue as we age; we either maintain what we have, or it recedes. As it recedes, the tooth appears to get longer in the mouth; this is the same with a natural tooth or with an implant. If there's recession, you may see the margin or the edge of the crown where it rests on the implant or on the root surface, and that can be unsightly, particularly on a front tooth. In the back of the mouth, it's actually almost an advantage, because then the patient can get in and clean around the tooth better.

It's important to remember that man-made teeth need to be maintained just like natural teeth. In fact, we recommend fluoride for our teen and adult patients who have crowns that rest right at the gumline or below because that junction between man-made material and tooth is the weakest part of any restoration in the mouth. Fluoride helps strengthen the tooth structure and fights against decay. We do a fluoride treatment at a cleaning appointment, and then we send it home with the patient to use during their normal maintenance routine of brushing, flossing, and using a water pick.

The fluoride treatment we currently use in the office is brushed on. We clean and dry the teeth, and then we brush it on and ask the patient not to eat or drink anything for a period of time. The longer it stays on the teeth, the better the uptake into the tooth structure.

There are different products that we send home with the patient to improve the appearance of teeth. One of these rebuilds the tooth on the molecular level; this is good for patients who have white blotches on their teeth resulting from poor cleaning around the brackets while wearing braces. Those blotches are decalcified areas that, in the office, we can eliminate with a slow-speed handpiece equipped with a rubber cup that essentially forces the fluoride into the enamel.

We also see decalcification at the gumline; this is where plaque loves to sit and where breakdown of the enamel occurs. It's not classified as decay because it hasn't broken through the enamel, but the enamel is so much weaker when we see this.

Gum Contouring

Gum contouring is sometimes a necessity when placing crowns, but other times it's a key cosmetic consideration.

For example, if while removing decay when prepping the tooth for a crown we had to go below the gum tissue more than normal, and if there is too much gum tissue above the margin of the prep, then we may not get a good impression. So we'll contour that gum tissue so we can capture a good impression but also so it'll be easier for the patient to clean around the crown.

We do it to create access for the dentist while having the crown made but also for the patient to be able to maintain the crown so it'll last longer.

We use a laser diode to remove gum tissue; the laser cuts and cauterizes at the same time, which means there's no bleeding, less inflammation, and rapid healing.

We also use it to perform frenectomy procedures, which is the removal of the frenum (the "tether" of tissue on the front lower or upper gum between the front of the teeth and the lip). Some people have a frenum that is too fibrous or too long, which can restrict lip movement, cause recession issues, or in some cases, create a space between the front two teeth. We see recession due to frenums more on the bottom than on the top, because there it gets pulled too much and is very thin, which can create periodontal problems.

Gum contouring is also used to help correct a crooked smile. For example, we can use it to sculpt a gum that is covering a front tooth and causing it to appear as though the neighboring tooth is longer. This is not unhealthy but just a little unsightly, as it's not symmetrical. We can sculpt that gum tissue so that the arch that the tissue makes around the tooth matches the tooth next to it.

The patient is numbed for contouring, so there's no discomfort during the procedure. If a lot of tissue is removed, there can be some soreness afterward, even though the gum is cauterized. Normally when we're sculpting tissue for cosmetic reasons, we only remove a small amount. But recovery from gum contouring typically takes up to 24 hours, and we tell patients to watch what they eat—avoiding acidic foods such as tomato sauce or orange juice—for a couple of meals following the procedure. Any discomfort can be handled with over-the-counter pain relievers.

Well-Designed Dentures Can Turn Back the Clock

Dentures of today can be designed with a younger appearance in mind. It's not about just putting teeth where teeth are missing; it's helping support facial features and muscles in the face, the mouth, and the lips.

Sometimes you might see someone who's wearing a denture, and you can tell it's a denture because it's too small—it doesn't support the face, so the face is collapsed. Or you'll see someone who looks like they're almost holding their breath—where there's way too much denture in the mouth.

That's why we don't just send in the impression to the lab, we send in as much information as possible. And when we get the denture back, if it's too thick in an area and it's pushing the patient's face out, we'll adjust the thickness to create a better look and fit. We can do that in the office.

However, when a patient has gone any length of time without teeth, new dentures can feel bulky at the start. So a lot of times a patient will have to get over that initial period of dealing with the bulk in the mouth. That's something we try to address on the front end before any impressions are made, during the treatment plan phase, because an upper denture covers the entire roof of the mouth—that's a huge change.

Also, the length of the teeth directly affects the way a denture looks in the mouth. Teeth that are too short age a person. We can design dentures so that the teeth are or appear to be longer so that there's more tooth showing below the lip line. Another factor is the color of the teeth; a lighter-colored tooth is a more youthful look because our tooth structure is stained more as we get older.

We can also design a denture so that the gum tissue looks very healthy.

When a patient comes to us in need of a denture replacement and they're already having problems that go beyond appearance because of ill-fitting dentures or just longtime wear and tear, then we can redesign dentures for them that not only fit and function better but that also have good esthetics.

Patients who are unhappy with their current dentures should see what's new; there is no need to keep wearing loose-fitting dentures that threaten to fall out, make it difficult to chew, or simply make you look old.

AT-HOME CARE FOR RESTORATIVE DENTISTRY

If you have been through restorative dentistry, then you'll want to take extra care at home to keep your teeth and mouth beautiful and functional for the long term.

DENTURES

Dentures can pick up stains and odors from food particles. They tend to get a little rough over time, especially on the teeth, which makes it easier for them to pick up stains.

We clean them in the office for patients, but there are also ways for them to be kept clean and sanitized at home.

The simplest way is to soak them at night using some of the over-the-counter tablets available for that purpose. Please note: household bleach is not an appropriate or safe denture cleaner, and other substances, such as Listerine mouthwash, can turn dentures colors.

After removing dentures from your mouth and before soaking them, you need to at least rinse them off. Ideally, you should clean them with a brush. There is a denture brush available—a very soft-bristled brush that is larger than a regular toothbrush. You can also use a toothbrush to clean dentures.

Anytime teeth are removed, the bone and tissue continues to resorb, affecting the fit of the denture over time. As the denture starts to become a little loose or just not fit as well, it will get to a point where it's time to refit or replace the denture.

Be sure to visit your dentist if your dentures don't fit properly. An ill-fitting denture can cause gum problems, which can lead to mouth sores and ultimately to oral cancer. If it's a partial denture, we recommend a visit to the dentist every six months. For patients with full dentures—at least once a year.

The majority of dentures are made of acrylic, which can wear down at a pretty quick pace. As your bite changes, you can develop symptoms of TMD.

CROWNS, BRIDGES, AND IMPLANTS

Cleaning crowns, bridges, and implants is similar to cleaning natural teeth. These restorations need to brushed and flossed, just as the other teeth in your mouth.

Some patients neglect flossing around crowns, believing that the crown acts as armor to keep decay from entering the tooth. But crowns mount onto underlying tooth structure, so they still need to be cleaned just like other teeth in the mouth.

Implants need a little extra attention. Although there is not any tooth structure involved with an implant, the gum tissue and bone around the implant must be kept clean to remain healthy. Since the bridge creates just that—a bridge—between teeth, it's important for patients to floss underneath the bridge and to clean between the anchored tooth and the natural tooth. Some patients rely on floss threaders to get floss into the space. But many patients turn to a Waterpik for that purpose because they can angle the tip under the bridge and flush that area out.

Chapter Five

FACIAL REJUVENATION: BEGINNING WITH BOTOX

The total transformation practice model is grounded in dental techniques that enhance oral health and appearance. But what makes this model truly unique is the facial rejuvenation techniques that build on that dental foundation to provide patients with a facial appearance that matches the beauty of their smile.

Total facial rejuvenation frames and restores the whole face, not just the teeth. Just as a smile is important to the total facial appearance, that total facial appearance is an important adjunct to the beauty of the smile.

As much as we've learned in our dental training, we've learned easily as much from the patients we treat. In fact, it was listening to them that lead us to develop this two-pronged model. Even when our patients' teeth were restored to a state that they could be proud of, they were still dissatisfied with wrinkles, creases, or other aspects of their facial appearance; their youthful smiles were actually making the rest of their face look older by comparison.

We often deal with lines on the lower face, such as lines on the corners of the mouth (the real ager is a drooping mouth).

But our facial rejuvenation is always done in comparison to a patient's aging. For instance, we don't give a 60-year-old patient lips like she had when she was 20. We've all seen that in magazines, and it doesn't look right. We don't turn back the clock that far; we're trying to enhance the beauty that the patient already has. We want to give her a natural look.

Sometimes a patient brings us a magazine and tells us she wants to look like the model in a picture. But the patient doesn't look anything like the model, so that's when we have to ask what the patient is really looking for: Does she really want to look like the model, or does she want what that person stands for?

Our Botox treatments gradually reverse the look of aging. Our approach is to use a very minimal dosage because the result we want is a more natural look, not a frozen face. We also want the patient to be happy with the result while getting used to the treatment.

As the Botox bonds to the muscles for the 90-day period that the treatment lasts, we want to see how that patient's body reacts to it because people heal at different rates. Patients' bodies react to anything we put in at different rates; for example, for some, anesthetic may last an hour and a half, and for others, it may last 45 minutes.

The best compliment we get with facial rejuvenation is when a patient comes back and says, "The people I work with keep saying to me, 'You look different. You look good. I can't tell what you've done.' Or they keep guessing, 'Did you get a new hairstyle? Did you change the color? Have you lost weight?'" And the patient doesn't tell anyone about the Botox or the Juvéderm, but people are noticing the difference for the better. They just can't say, "Oh, you've had all that done to your face."

In the total facial appearance arena, we have an advantage because we understand how to extend the sensitivity and sensibility of technical dental perfection to facial rejuvenation. For example, we could give a patient dentures that are technically perfect but look fake in the mouth. We know how to make those teeth perfect for the patient.

It's the same with facial rejuvenation. We're just trying to help patients look as healthy as they can. Again, that goes back to actually being healthy more than anything else. But if you look better and if you're feeling better about yourself, it lends to health.

BOTOX: THE BRIDGE BETWEEN DENTISTRY AND FACIAL REJUVENATION

In 2012, the Georgia Board of Dentistry voted to allow dentists to deliver Botox, and we were in the second group of dentists to take the course.

When we first started in dentistry, Botox was a frontline defense for pain management with TMD because it binds to the muscle and prevents it from completely contracting and moving the way it normally does. At that time, physicians saw what else it did with facial esthetics. For instance, if a person frowned or scrunched up his eyebrows, between the eyebrows he had creases that ran vertically; usually it's two creases, and we call that "the 11." A patient can get these creases when they are dealing with pain and are constantly grimacing because of the discomfort. Botox helps to relax the muscles that create the creases.

At the same time, patients were seeing other results that they really liked—such as the smoothing out of frown creases—after receiving Botox for help with the pain resulting from clenching. Helping the pain areas relax also helped with other facial features.

That's how Botox landed in the realm of dentistry: dentists saw advantages of it initially with pain management, although it wasn't approved by the Food and Drug Administration for treating migraines until 2010. The two uses, relief of pain from clenching and migraine headaches, go hand in hand because Botox binds to the muscle, so it's affecting how that muscle works. It treats the muscle below the skin, which affects the wrinkles on the skin. And the movement of the muscle—the expansion and contraction—is actually causing the pain and causing the wrinkles.

While Botox is considered the first line of defense for TMD, it's not the cure-all; TMD also involves bone, cartilage, and nerves, so Botox strictly helps diagnose and treat the muscular piece of the problem. Its application in TMD is to prevent those contractions and spasms of the muscle that put pressure on the associated structures and the nerve, thereby causing pain. Reducing the contraction of the muscles helps disseminate stress and pressure to other surrounding structures.

We use a very precise, low dose of Botox to alter the contraction of the muscle; we don't want to paralyze the muscle or completely take away its function. We don't want to give patients a frozen face; we want them to have expression—to have facial movement.

Again, it's because of our methods that we think we're the best qualified to do these treatments.

We also maintain detailed documentation—every time we make an injection, we know exactly where we put it. We use an eyebrow pencil to make small marks of the exact injection sites, and then we take a picture of those marks. That goes in the patient's chart, so the next time she comes in we know exactly where we injected the Botox last time. If we got the results we wanted out of the previous injection, then we go back in the exact same areas. Or, if we want to alter the results, then we change some areas.

But again, our goal is always to just reduce the contractile force on the muscle; we only want to restrict the muscle somewhat, not take it out of commission. For a natural and pleasing appearance, the muscles of the face still need to function, so we don't want to administer Botox to the point of immobilization of the muscles. We want patients to be able to show expressions and to laugh and smile and show those pretty teeth we just restored.

HOW TREATMENT WORKS

We treat three areas on the upper face. One is the forehead, or the frontalis muscle, which is what causes the furrows in the forehead. Then there's the glabellar complex, which includes the procerus muscle between the eyebrows and the corrugator muscles above the eyebrows; these are what cause the "11" lines or the "H" between the eyes. And then there are the crow's feet, or the orbicularis oculi, which are the round muscles that circle the eyes. This group of muscles in the upper face can be the cause of migraine headaches.

In treating these areas, we use a syringe with a very fine needle. It's actually an insulin syringe, which, because of our family's history with diabetes, is something we're very accustomed to handling.

As far as dosage amounts, we don't rely on a "cookbook," we look at these specific areas on the face on each particular patient, decide our dosage, and then do the injections based on the dosage we deem appropriate. It's not a rubber-stamp process; we don't decide that every patient is going to get the same amount of units.

However, for esthetics treatments, the initial dosage we use with every patient is very minimal; it's typically much less per site than the amount used for the TMD application.

Early Botox treatments wear off in about three months; the body completely metabolizes it. Many tell us at the three-month point that the treatment seems to have worn off or that the muscles are reverting to the state they were in when we started treatment. But after a few treatments of Botox done every three months, the muscles seem to "retrain" themselves to contract by a certain amount for that period of time; at that point, the patient can possibly go four months between treatments.

It's similar to someone retraining their muscles through regular exercise. If they stretch their hamstring every day, then that muscle gets used to being stretched to that particular length. Facial muscles react in the same way. If we inject Botox to bind to a muscle to only allow it to contract to a certain level, then the muscle gets used to that. So it's not that the Botox is wearing off more slowly, but rather, the results are lasting longer because of retraining.

Botox and Juvéderm are ideal for patients from ages 28 to 65. And on the esthetic side, that's really the people we're seeing: the people who are active when they're younger and who continue to remain active because it's on their minds tend to stay healthy and to look their best. They're more health conscious and more proactive about their health, rather than just saying, "I don't work out like I used to. Everybody gets old."

But we're very discrete about the treatments also because we've found that many patients don't want even their immediate family members to know they're receiving Botox or Juvéderm. They just want to enhance their appearance.

As for the pain during the treatment, it's a little like plucking an eyebrow; it's really not painful at all. We use multiple syringes during a treatment so that we're not delivering the Botox with a dull needle. We use a different syringe for each area that we're treating; that's the key to the painless injection aspect of the treatment.

As with any treatment of the skin, there can be some redness in the area of the injection site. It's a little like a mosquito bite—there's some initial skin irritation, but it's very short-lived. Sometimes the redness is gone by the time we've completed the checkout paperwork.

Once in a while we'll see a little bruising, but in general that's pretty minor, and it can be concealed with makeup.

And because it can take a little time for the material to actually bind to the muscle, we tell all of our new patients after we've injected the initial Botox treatment that we don't want them to love it or hate it for 10 to 14 days.

That's one reason why we ask patients to return two weeks after the injection. We ask them to come back so that we can check the results and do a touch-up dose, if needed. This is how we determine if an amount needs to be added to the dosage. Often, nothing else needs to be done, but we like them to come back so that we can see the results and make sure the patient is pleased with the results.

Earlier in the book we talked a little about how we treat gummy smiles. This is when a patient shows too much gum tissue when they smile. We're seeing great results in treating this condition with Botox.

In the past, a gummy smile had to be treated with surgery; it required breaking the maxilla (the bone in the upper portion of the jaw). Now, it's a much easier procedure requiring injections in two different areas with Botox. This relaxes the muscle that raises the lip. The patient can still smile, laugh, and show expression; it's just that the upper lip will not rise as high when the patient moves their mouth.

Repairing a gummy smile epitomizes the bridge between Botox for dental procedures, such as TMD, and Botox for facial rejuvenation.

We also use Botox to treat "smoker's lines" around the mouth. When treating this area with Botox, we usually recommend a combination of treatments. Botox relaxes the muscle that circles the mouth, but our esthetician also recommends doing chemical peels and CIT, or collagen induction therapy treatments.

Medical-Grade Botox

There is a lot of news today about Botox coming from outside the United States.

In our practice, we only use Botox that we order direct from the maker, which is Allergan. This allows us to deliver predictable and reliable results with medical-grade quality. Botox comes in a form that has to be reconstituted into a liquid form, but we strictly follow the guidelines of the American Academy of Facial Esthetics, which is what the maker recommends. That's how we get the predictable results of the injections lasting 90 days. Greater dilution will still allow the Botox to bind to the muscle, but by following the recommended ratio, we can better predict what it's going to do.

In 2012, the Georgia Board of Dentistry approved the use of Botox by dentists who have completed a board-approved post-doctoral course in administering the injectable pharmacologic. We were among the first to take the course (in the second class)—so early in the game, in fact, that we were in class with members of the board of dentistry.

The courses we took for Botox included use of it for both pain management and esthetics. At the time, we also took courses on dermal fillers, and we remain students of the American Academy of Facial Esthetics as part of our continuing education for dentistry.

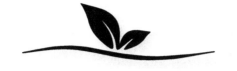

Chapter Six

DERMAL FILLERS: FINE-TUNING FACIAL CONTOURS AND APPEARANCE

While Botox yields remarkable results when it comes to erasing signs of aging, such as laugh lines, crow's feet, and forehead wrinkles, those features aren't the only things that age the face.

Collagen is responsible for giving the face a plump, youthful appearance; it is the "pillowy" support beneath the skin that is lost naturally over time. This loss is accelerated by factors like sun exposure and smoking, which can leave the face looking hollowed-out and drawn. Combined with a loss of elastin—the intertwined fibrous proteins in skin that support it and keep it tight, yet flexible—skin on the face begins to form creases and visible lines. These creases and lines form on the face due to the actions of muscles that can't be immobilized by Botox.

Think of elastin as fine fibers that intertwine and support the cells of the skin. When those fibers break down, they sag—that's what causes the creasing in the skin. Also, when moisture loss occurs and the collagen is lost, that also breaks down the skin cells and causes sagging.

So collagen plumps up the cells of the facial skin, and elastin helps support those cells. And while we want to preserve as much collagen and elastin as we possibly can, fillers can help rejuvenate areas where elastin is lagging. Botox is not appropriate for these areas, because these muscles control the movements of the mouth.

These special, facial agers are the reason that we offer dermal fillers as another tool in our arsenal of rejuvenation techniques.

HOW DO DERMAL FILLERS WORK?

The dermal filler that we use is a hyaluronic acid, a matrix-like substance that retains moisture.

Sometimes called liquid facelifts, dermal fillers are nonsurgical options commonly used to restore the youthful contours of the lips and face.

In our practice, we use dermal fillers to correct the nasolabial folds, which run from the base of the nose down to the corner of the lips, and "marionette lines," which are the turned-down corners of the mouth.

The filler is injected into the dermis—the underlying area just below the surface of the skin—and gives immediate support where it's been lost in the lower features of the face.

Another area we use filler is what we call a "black triangle," which is when someone has lost gum tissue between the two front teeth resulting in a space that looks like a black triangle. We inject the filler into this area, and it plumps up the gum and immediately fills the space.

Our office uses Juvéderm, which also contains Lidocaine, a numbing agent that helps with comfort at the injection site. Juvéderm has been around for a long time, so it has a proven safety and efficacy profile. A dermal filler treatment lasts 9 to 12 months.

Often, we perform dermal filler procedures for patients after they've had a dental cleaning or restoration—when they mention that they don't like the "smile lines" around their mouth.

We start the procedure by numbing the patient just as we would for a dental procedure; we begin with an injection inside the mouth. We follow that with an injection of the Juvéderm on the face, through the surface of the skin into the dermal layer. We use a threading technique, which is just laying down several thin threads of the material where the fold or wrinkle is. Depending on the depth of the fold, we may lay down up to three threads of the material. Again, one benefit of using Juvéderm is that it contains the numbing agent Lidocaine.

Another plus of Juvéderm is that the results are immediate. With Botox, the results take 10 to 14 days to materialize. With Juvéderm, the patient sees the results as soon as they leave the office; it's immediate gratification for younger-looking skin.

The whole procedure—to do one area, such as both of the nasolabial folds—takes around 45 minutes from start to finish.

We often do dermal fillers in conjunction with a dental procedure, since the patient is already numb. For example, if a patient was getting a filling or crown done on the upper arch, that area would already be numb because of the dental procedure, and a dermal filler procedure would add another 30 minutes or so to the patient's time in the chair. Patients who have dermal filler procedures performed often have Botox done as well.

Like the Botox, the dermal fillers procedure makes a noticeable difference—not so much that a procedure has been done but that the patient looks different. Typically, what we hear from patients is that people tell them that they look refreshed—like they've been on vacation.

WHY WE ARE MORE

Spa services are also offered at Total Transformation Dental and Spa. Painted a tranquil shade of blue, our spa room is filled with soothing music and candles that offer a very calming environment for amenities that relax and pamper our clients. Services are performed by our licensed esthetician, Rhonda Castro, who has been with the practice for more than 15 years.

At Total Transformation Dental and Spa, we believe healthy skin is influenced by many factors, including heredity, sun protection, and the environment. The way you take care of your skin will directly influence the way it looks years from now when the damage you've done finally shows. So a good skin care routine is a key factor in helping to slow the aging process and to eliminate problems before they begin. This includes getting facials, peels, and using professional skin care products for your particular skin type.

WHY PROFESSIONAL GRADE SKIN CARE RATHER THAN OVER-THE-COUNTER PRODUCTS?

The active ingredients in professional skin care products are much stronger, more potent, and of much better quality. Because they are so much more effective, you will see significant results that will also save you money. Over-the-counter products tend to use harsh cleansers that strip the natural oil barrier. This causes your skin to be drier and appear dull. It may also cause the skin to overproduce more oil to counteract this unbalanced condition, which in turn causes clogged pores and acne.

Furthermore, most over-the-counter scrubs have large, abrasive particles that actually stretch the pores and cause tiny tears or abrasions in the skin. Also, if you have ever turned the bottle or container around and taken a good look at the ingredients listed, you would see that a lot of them are suspect and contain harsh chemicals and parabens, which are designed to greatly prolong the shelf life of many products. For the above reasons, we trust, use, and recommend the professional skin care line Image Skincare.

We recommend daily use of good, professional skin care products at home, morning and evening, for beautiful skin. In the morning, your skin is cleansed and prepared for the day, while the evening cleanse optimizes the skin to restore and repair during the night. We also advise implementing exfoliation into your routine at least twice per week with a facial scrub brush or a good clay masque.

Regular use of sunscreen is also an important part of your daily skin care regimen, and we're very passionate about sharing that. Although Americans spend about $1 billion annually on sunscreen products, half say they skip it. We should aim for a broad-spectrum sunscreen that protects against both UVA and UVB rays. Make sure it's SPF 30–50 and water resistant up to 80 minutes—no sunscreen is waterproof. The bottom line: sunscreen helps to prevent wrinkles, prevent age spots, and ward off skin cancers by forming a protective barrier that blocks UVA and UVB rays. Every time you tan or burn, you damage your skin, speeding up the aging process and increasing your risk of skin cancers. There is no safe way to suntan—*ever*.

According to the Skin Cancer Foundation, more than 90 percent of the visible changes commonly attributed to skin aging are caused by the sun. This is a very doable step. We just have to open those bottles of sunscreen we're all purchasing but not using! Sunscreen should be applied to all exposed areas when outdoors including the décolletage, backs of hands, neck, ears, and top of the head, if you are bald.

SPA SERVICES

Our spa services include various types of facials. We offer a Short and Sweet Facial, great for when you need a little pick me up or great for teens just being introduced to the importance of a good skin care routine.

For normal skin, our Look Great Feel Great Facial is an amazing, one-hour facial that includes a face-and-scalp massage—a very relaxing experience.

We offer facials for men, too! Men tend to just wash their face with soap, and they are also outside a lot. Because of this, their skin tends to be on the dry side. The Maintain Your Man Card Facial is a refining facial that will leave rough, dry skin feeling clean, soothed, and refreshed. It's great for de-stressing too.

Facials for normal skin are recommended once per month to maintain and keep beautiful skin.

We also perform specialty facials designed to address specific skin care concerns from acne-blemish control to anti-aging or dehydration. Oily or acneic skin requires a more careful approach to balance this condition. We recommend both a facial and a peel once per week.

Aging skin, or problematic skin such as hyperpigmentation, needs a more aggressive approach. As we age, the normal skin cell turnover process slows down significantly. In order to speed up the cell turnover and reveal the newer, plumper cells underneath, we recommend a monthly peel session for five to ten months along with a once monthly facial. Once the desired results are achieved, a glycolic acid peel is administered once every three months.

Our free consultation can help design the perfect skin care routine for you. As mentioned above, chemical peels are yet another popular service we offer.

A peel is a chemical exfoliation process that removes and buffs away the dead skin cells on the outer layer that we see. Fruit enzyme peels are great peels for this purpose because they are so gentle to the skin and yet are still able to really give the skin a polished glow. We have a great fruit enzyme peel called the O2 Lift. This is a safe and effective treatment that offers all the benefits of a chemical peel without the redness, flaking, and peeling. It is so gentle, no one will ever know you've had a peel, but they will ask you why you look so refreshed.

Glycolic or retinol peels get a little deeper, penetrating the outer layer to diminish fine lines, wrinkles, and uneven skin tone. Glycolic peels are also a great benefit for the neck area and the top of the hands where we tend to see other signs of aging.

Need smoker's lines and deeper wrinkles treated? Our Jessner's peel is a specialty peel for treatment of severely damaged skin due to smoking and extreme sun exposure. This peel penetrates deeply, causing generous peeling for three to five days, treating advanced face aging concerns.

Because the skin is vulnerable after any peel treatment, all chemical peel skin care clients leave with a post peel treatment kit that provides skin-calming nutrients and protection during this delicate repair period. Peels are recommended once monthly for problematic skin care concerns or once a season for normal skin.

We also perform CIT treatments. This skin-rejuvenating treatment stimulates the body's own collagen production in the dermal layer by way of collagen induction therapy, also called micro-needling. It works by introducing a series of very fine, sharp needles into the skin following the administration of a medical-grade topical anesthetic to reduce discomfort. The needles are moved over the surface of the skin to create microscopic channels or columns at various depths. This creates micro-damage to the dermis, thereby encouraging the body to repair and generate new cells that form the collagen and elastin fibers. It reduces the appearance of fine lines, wrinkles, stretch marks, acne scarring, skin laxity, age spots, and cellulite. It also greatly enhances the skin's appearance by channeling ingredients such as vitamin C and hyaluronic acid deeper into the dermal layers to maximize effectiveness. Although it is performed primarily on the face, it can be performed anywhere on the body.

Other services on our spa menu include waxing and eyebrow and eyelash tinting. We also offer eyelash extensions, including Classic, Silk, and Mink single-lash extensions. Our Luscious Lashes tier packages include a full set plus one free full refill monthly for 12 months. Eyelash extensions are a great way to look and feel glamorous all the time.

Esthetician services are offered during normal office hours, and the services can be booked to take place following a dental procedure or as a standalone treatment. In fact, many patients have a facial or other esthetic services done after a crown or a filling, which works out quite well because it is a very relaxing way to end an appointment that patients really enjoy.

Facial Rejuvenation: The Importance of At-Home Skincare

Part of our facial rejuvenation procedures includes education on how you can maintain and optimize your look once you've left the office.

As mentioned previously, we recommend daily use of good, professional skincare products at home—morning and evening—for beautiful and healthy skin.

Regular use of sunscreen is also an important part of a skincare regimen. The sun is the biggest skin ager, so sunscreen needs to be incorporated in with other products that are used. Having sunscreen in your foundation makeup is not enough; at least a 30 SPF sunscreen really needs to be applied every morning. Any sunscreen is better than nothing, but we offer products that complement one another.

Sunscreen should also be applied to the chest area, the décolletage area, and to the backs of hands.

Any woman who's interested in enhancing her appearance and fighting the signs of aging probably has a closet full of products. But many just don't know what order to use them in. Our esthetic services can cut through the confusion and help you make sense of what you need.

We use the Image product line, which includes three products in the morning (a cleanser, a moisturizer, and a sunscreen), and two in the evening (a cleanser and a heavier moisturizer designed to protect and repair the skin). For the morning application, we tell clients to mix the moisturizer and sunscreen in the morning, which cuts down on one step, and then let that set a minute before applying makeup. The evening routine is just to cleanse again and then put on the evening moisturizer. Then twice a week, we suggest a mask or scrub to clear pores and exfoliate to remove dead skin. This helps the moisturizer penetrate more deeply into the skin because it's not fighting through all that dead skin.

If a client already has products that they love, we recommend that they stick with those, and then we may offer some of our products to treat specific needs or to complement what they're already using.

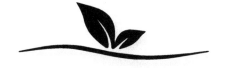

Chapter Seven

TOTAL TRANSFORMATION: SEE FOR YOURSELF

A total transformation at Total Transformation Dental and Spa usually starts with the patient wanting a change. It might be dental treatment for a pain-related problem, or it might be that they don't like the way a tooth looks; because of our esthetic focus, we don't just fix teeth—we also make them attractive. So whether it's decay that ultimately requires a crown or a crooked tooth that needs a veneer, we have the expertise to resolve these problems of the mouth.

Our goal is to have each patient's teeth and mouth not only restore well and function soundly but also look nice and be something the patient is happy with and proud of.

Once the patient is smiling again, they typically start looking at other areas to improve. A beautiful, pain-free smile changes the whole demeanor; when they have something they're proud of when smiling and talking, it changes their confidence level. It really changes their whole personality. That's when most patients decide they want to make even more of an investment in their appearance.

PATIENT #1 (BILL)

When Bill came to Total Transformation Dental and Spa, his problems were both comfort and esthetics.

His front two teeth had root canals in the past, but the teeth had never been restored, so he was embarrassed by how they looked.

One of his front teeth was discolored and had a broken edge, and it was a real issue for him when he smiled. So he didn't smile. His gums were in generally good health, although he had some decay issues. But if we didn't address the restoration of those two teeth, we were going to lose them. The root canals had been done, but he'd lost the temporary fillings that had been placed on the backside of those teeth, so basically anything that was going in his mouth was running the risk of damaging the root canals.

He was so self-conscious about the look of his smile that it reflected on his demeanor and made him less effective at the work he did. He worked with people every day and was especially involved with teenagers.

When he first came in, he was very embarrassed about how everything looked; he didn't even really want us to look or get started. He wasn't necessarily concerned about pain or going through something uncomfortable because he'd had dental work in the past. It wasn't a bad experience; it was just that he hadn't done it in a while.

He was also a little concerned about the amount of time it would take to fix his problems. Since he had a young family, he tended to put himself last on the list of priorities, so by the time he came to us, he was at the point where he knew he had to do something. He didn't know that he had almost waited too long; he just wanted to know what his options were. At the time, he was 30 years old, but his teeth made him look at least a decade older.

At the urging of his wife and mother-in-law, he finally came to see us.

First, we had to address all his concerns about his appearance and the time it would take. But once we got past those issues and we made him comfortable with us and his surroundings, we were able to deal with his teeth.

Our first concern was whether the two front teeth would be strong enough to hold individual restorations themselves. Whenever you are dealing with a root canal, the nerves are out of the tooth so there's no more blood supply or nutrients running to the inside of the tooth, and it can definitely become brittle. We told him that was always an issue with these teeth, especially the length of time involved since the root canals had been done.

Ultimately, we put posts in the two teeth to stabilize them, and then we did the core buildup, which is rebuilding the solid part of the inside of the tooth to attach the crown. Then we took an impression of all six of the front teeth and fabricated temporary crowns for them to make sure that they were in a solid state and everything was stable.

Those temporaries served as sort of a preview of what was to come, which made a complete difference in Bill at that early point in time.

It gave him a sense of confidence almost immediately that he was going in the right direction with his teeth.

We rechecked his temporaries after six weeks, and everything was still stable. So we impressed for the permanent crowns, put the temporaries back on, and sent the impression to the lab. It takes two and a half to three weeks to get the crowns back from the lab, so Bill came back for another appointment later, and we removed the temporary crowns and cemented in the permanent ones.

Afterward, Bill became a different person, and the change was immediate. From the moment he left the office, he couldn't get over how he looked. You can see the difference in the second two photos of his before-and-after smile. His smile is not only broader, but it's a lot more relaxed. Just from this partial-face photo, you can see that he is happy rather than self-conscious.

The photos also show how he got back the length of the teeth and the edges; he got back close to what he had before. That can help a patient speak better, and it improves phonetics. Especially with what he does for a living, being in front of people and talking with them constantly, it put him more at ease. He didn't have to watch how he smiled or laughed because he was embarrassed of how the teeth looked. It really just loosened him up more.

After he had the work done, the teens he worked with commented repeatedly on how much more he smiled. To get a teenager to recognize that—well, it really boosted his confidence. They basically told him, "You're a different person."

And it wasn't just the teenagers. His wife, his mother-in-law, and everybody that came in contact with him could see the difference that the changes in his mouth made—not only in his smile but also in his confidence. It changed him overall as a person.

When he first came in, Bill really seemed a little beaten down. But now he carries himself differently.

He's definitely more comfortable with himself, but he's also more comfortable with us. At first, it seemed like he thought we were going to judge him or chastise him for not having something done sooner.

So now he's comfortable coming in here, and that is a huge plus when doing the type of transformation that he went through or when just maintaining a healthy mouth.

As the patient, you want to be comfortable where you're going for your treatment. You sit in the biggest, most intimidating chair in the room, so in our practice, it's important for that comfort level to be there first. That's what builds the trust.

Now Bill comes in for his regular appointments because we impress on him the importance of protecting his investment. That's true in all phases of dentistry. It's not a one shot and everything's done; you have to follow up with maintenance.

PATIENT #2 (MELISSA KAO, TREATMENT COORDINATOR)

Melissa Kao, treatment coordinator at Total Transformation Dental and Spa, had a number of issues resolved by the practice.

Kao had issues with breaking teeth and with her TMJ. Her transformation was for both esthetics and functionality.

Her issues started when she had three root canals with crowns, side by side, on the upper right side of her mouth over a period of about four months. The problem was not caused by decay; it was the result of clenching and grinding. Kao would clench and grind her teeth to the point where she would crack a tooth, thereby exposing a nerve.

Sometime later, she started experiencing the same problem in other areas of her mouth.

At that point, we recommended crowning 20 of Kao's teeth to change how everything fit together inside her mouth. In this way, if her clenching broke something, it would break porcelain, not natural teeth.

Kao found the solution to her liking; she had already had adult braces twice and still had orthodontic issues afterward. Restoring her teeth eliminated the clenching and grinding issues as well as the cosmetic and orthodontic issues. "We killed three birds with one stone," she says.

The amount of damage being done inside Kao's mouth, along with the three existing root canals, dictated her teeth being restored right away to prevent more damage.

Total restoration of her mouth took eight years to complete. Of the original round, Kao has had a couple of premolars replaced—the teeth that absorb the most pressure—with state-of-the-art material designed specifically for people who clench and grind. But the front teeth that she smiles with have remained intact since they were replaced in 2007.

The original procedures involved getting like materials opposing each other. Porcelain is much harder than enamel, so if a severe clencher or grinder has porcelain clenching against natural tooth structure, it will wear away the enamel very fast. So a big piece of Kao's treatment was getting a good comfortable bite with like materials chewing together, so that when she closed her teeth together, further wear would be prevented. We were trying to even things out so we would have equal pressure on both sides; we needed the back teeth to be able to take compression forces that we put them under. That also helps position the front teeth, which are smaller, thinner, and tend to wear faster.

Doing crowns in a larger series gave us the advantage of being able to balance the bite effectively, rather than just going tooth by tooth.

Also, by fixing the front six or eight teeth at a time, the same batch of porcelain can be used to get a more symmetrical look. It's like buying rolls of wallpaper, which is made in batches—the same pattern made a few months later could easily have subtle differences.

Without the treatment, Kao would have undoubtedly continued to require root canals, and—worse—had she succeeded in splitting a tooth, it would have had to be removed.

Kao says having everything lined up in the mouth evened out the pressures throughout the mouth and cut down on the sensitivity, making chewing and eating more comfortable.

For Kao, restoration was a better choice over appliances because appliances only serve as a buffer between the teeth to slow down damage tooth to tooth. When the appliance is in the mouth and the teeth cannot come together all the way, the muscles that contract when they close are not contracting all the way. Those muscles are being retrained to only contract a certain amount.

So appliances work while they are in, which is usually at night when most "bruxers," as they are called, tend to clench and grind their teeth. But very rarely does the clenching and grinding problem completely go away unless the circumstances around it change. Clenching is caused by a number of factors: sometimes that's a change in jobs, a change in marital status, or a change in economic status. It's not all just a tooth issue.

Restoration was also chosen because Kao had chewed through some of the best appliances available and still broke teeth. Her teeth were in danger, and she needed a solution. That solution not only resolved her structural issues but also gave her a stunning smile.

"It's a huge weight off your shoulders when you're not walking around in pain from sensitivity," she says, adding that she no longer wakes up with grit in her mouth and having to face the dread of looking in the mirror to see where the break occurred.

She also has more confidence at work. Working in the dental industry, it was important for Kao to have teeth that look their best. Now she can tell patients firsthand about the experience. "I have patients tell me every day, 'I want my teeth to look like yours. Yours are absolutely beautiful,'" she says. And, she adds, patients are stunned when she tells them they are not her natural teeth. "I've been in the chair," she tells them.

Kao also decided to have Botox performed after we completed training. Although Kao is not allowed to administer Botox in the state of Georgia, she went through training because she has to constitute and pull the Botox for us to administer.

She had injections in her forehead and around her eyebrows and eyes and continues to have treatments regularly. Kao says the treatments make her feel good about herself, and once the wrinkles are gone, she doesn't want them to come back.

She also does them so she can look good for patients and so that she can tell them about her own experience. "When they say they're nervous about the Botox because they don't like needles, I show them where I have them done."

PATIENT #3
(DR. JULIE MARSHALL)

Dr. Julie Marshall is a prime example of what total transformation from Total Transformation Dental and Spa can achieve. As the daughter of a dentist and a dentist herself, she naturally had a good foundation of very healthy gums. Her problem was the shortening of the teeth that naturally occurs as a result of aging; in her mid-40s, she was experiencing a classic reverse smile.

Consequently, she wouldn't show a lot of teeth when she smiled, and working with people every day, she felt it important to look better, not only from a business standpoint but from a personal one also. Her case was a classic example of the patients that the practice is dedicated to.

So she wanted to get crowns to lengthen her teeth. She had eight anterior crowns done on her upper teeth, along with lightening, so that all of the top teeth matched and presented an even smile to the world.

Dr. Baxter performed the procedure.

He did all of the preliminary examinations and records, and there was minimal prepping involved. Plus it helped that the patient was open about her needs and wants.

Temporaries were still required because of the amount of time needed at the lab, but the total transformation took about three weeks from start to finish. There are no special favors at Baxter & Marshall; patients come first, so available time still had to be scheduled between the sibling performing the procedure and the sibling in the patient chair.

With esthetic dentistry, it's possible to have either a very "Hollywood" look or a very natural look. Marshall opted for the natural look, and most patients don't know she's had work done.

She was very pleased with the results and says she constantly receives comments on how pretty her teeth are. Marshall's experience allowed her to see firsthand what a transformation feels like and the personal fulfillment it gives.

Many patients request teeth that look like Dr. Marshall's: "We want teeth that look like yours," they'll tell us. And it's very easy for her to tell them what type of restoration she has, how long they've been in her mouth, and how she functions with them. It actually helps patients to see her teeth in action; it helps them decide if it's something they want for themselves.

With the esthetic dentistry complete, Marshall decided she wanted to do more to improve her appearance. Her smile gave her the confidence to take her appearance to the next level.

After the practice began facial esthetic procedures, Dr. Marshall decided to have some herself. Dr. Baxter administered Juvéderm injections in the lower face and also Botox to treat smoker's lines around the mouth.

She received her first treatment in December 2012 and has received injections every three months since.

"Because of my positive experiences, procedures, and work at Total Transformation Dental and Spa, I feel a lot better about myself. I'm more confident, and I want to pass that confidence on to others."

After the treatments, Marshall also started wearing false eyelashes to make up for a loss of lashes due to aging; it's something she says she never would have considered had her confidence not been boosted by the facial esthetic procedures.

These subtle enhancements make Marshall feel better about herself but also make her look younger. There's a real difference in her look, demeanor, and the way she carries herself today compared with a few years ago.

Marshall says that the excitement she and Kao feel about the facial esthetic procedures—how much they like them and what the injections are doing for them—comes through when they talk about them with patients. "It's easy to quote and to sell because patients can see how much we like doing it," Marshall says.

ABOUT THE AUTHORS

Drs. Marshall and Baxter continually further their education in cosmetic and restorative dentistry through professional memberships in the American Dental Association, Georgia Dental Association, Academy of Facial Esthetics, and the Academy of General Dentistry.

DR. JULIE MARSHALL

Julie B. Marshall, DMD, graduated from the Medical College of Georgia with a doctor of dental medicine degree in 1988. She currently practices general dentistry with an emphasis in family, restorative, and cosmetic care.

Dr. Marshall enjoys working with families in maintaining their oral health. She resides in Alpharetta with her husband Scott and two children.

DR. DOUG BAXTER

Doug P. Baxter, DMD, graduated from the Medical University of South Carolina with a doctor of dental medicine degree in 1992. He practices general dentistry with an emphasis on family, restorative, and cosmetic care.

Dr. Baxter enjoys providing dental services to the families that he has grown up with, as well as welcoming new families to the Winder community. He resides in Winder with his wife Shannon and three children.

OUR INVITATION

We invite you to learn more about our practice and the services we offer. Please visit our website: www.baxterandmarshall.com.

New patients are welcome. Insurance is filed for you, no-interest financing is available, and major credit cards are welcome.

Drs. Doug Baxter and Julie Marshall provide a full range of dental services to families in Winder, Georgia, and the surrounding Auburn, Carl, and Barrow County communities. We enjoy caring for entire families spanning multiple generations. Our doctors and team are dedicated to taking the time needed to provide the very best care to every patient of any age.

We are pleased to offer our patients the following services in a friendly and comfortable environment:

- Cosmetic dentistry
- Tooth-colored fillings
- Facial esthetics
- Laser dentistry
- Family dentistry
- Diabetes and oral care
- Lumineers
- Teeth whitening
- Porcelain veneers
- Metal-free crowns
- Invisalign
- Headache therapy
- Dental implants

- Dentures and partials
- TMJ
- Gum disease treatment
- Velscope